Theory of
Drug
Development

Chapman & Hall/CRC Biostatistics Series

Chapman & Hall/CRC Biostatistics Series

Chapman & Hall/CRC Biostatistics Series

Theory of Drug Development

Eric B. Holmgren

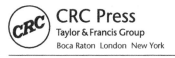

CRC Press
Taylor & Francis Group
Boca Raton London New York

CRC Press is an imprint of the
Taylor & Francis Group, an **informa** business

A CHAPMAN & HALL BOOK

CRC Press
Taylor & Francis Group
6000 Broken Sound Parkway NW, Suite 300
Boca Raton, FL 33487-2742

First issued in paperback 2018

© 2014 by Taylor & Francis Group, LLC
CRC Press is an imprint of Taylor & Francis Group, an Informa business

No claim to original U.S. Government works

ISBN-13: 978-1-4665-0746-3 (hbk)
ISBN-13: 978-1-138-37468-3 (pbk)

Library of Congress Cataloging-in-Publication Data

Holmgren, Eric B., 1959-
Theory of drug development / Eric B. Holmgren.
pages cm -- (Chapman & Hall/CRC biostatistics series)
"A CRC title."
Includes bibliographical references and index.
ISBN 978-1-4665-0746-3 (hardcover : alk. paper)
1. Drugs--Design. 2. Drug development. 3. Pharmaceutical industry. I. Title.

RM301.25.H65 2014
615.1'9--dc23   2013027620

Visit the Taylor & Francis Web site at
http://www.taylorandfrancis.com

and the CRC Press Web site at
http://www.crcpress.com

Contents

Section II   A Theory of Evidence in Drug Development

Section III Additional Topics

Preface

This book will provide the reader with a rationale for the practice of drug development, both from the perspective of a drug company as well as from the perspective of a regulatory agency. In many situations, the theory presented herein should facilitate an understanding of the current practice of drug development. However, in some cases the theory presented here may not exactly coincide with current practice and indeed may point to other ways of conducting or evaluating clinical trials. In either case, the quantitative foundation provided here will enable us to more systematically address issues that arise in drug development. Examples of such issues that are addressed in this book include the following: What is the impact of adaptive designs on the quality of drugs that receive marketing approval? How can we design a Phase 3 pivotal study that permits data-driven adjustment of the treatment effect estimate? When do we have enough information to know that a drug improves survival time for the whole patient population, not just the fraction of the patient experience represented by the amount of follow-up time in the study? We can start to approach problems like this in a systematic way once we have quantified many of the ideas underlying drug development, as has been done in this book.

The first part of this book concerns the efficient development of drugs and originated with an experience that occurred shortly after I started working in the pharmaceutical industry at Hoechst Roussel in Bridgewater, New Jersey. I was asked to determine the sample size for a Phase 2 trial, and after researching the literature to find a good estimate of the variance for the primary endpoint of the trial, I calculated how large the sample size had to be to provide 80 percent power with a type 1 error of 0.05. When I presented the numbers to the clinician I was working with at the time, she promptly said that the number was too big and stated what the size of the trial was going to be without doing any of the sample size calculations that I had done. No doubt this experience is shared by many other statisticians in the pharmaceutical industry when they were fresh out of a Ph.D. program in statistics. After recovering from this encounter with a clinician, I felt that there must be a quantitative explanation for designing Phase 2 trials with sample sizes that do not achieve 80 percent power and started thinking of formal rationales for smaller trials.

The origin of the second part of the book, which concerns evidence in drug development, occurred relatively recently while I was working on immunology products at Genentech. I was asked to look at a negative Phase 3 trial in an immunologic disease to see if there was any way it could be salvaged. The trial was sized to detect a hazard ratio of 0.6 and the estimated hazard ratio was coming in at 0.75, which in many circumstances could be considered clinically meaningful. It appeared that the drug had activity but that the trial was simply underpowered. I knew that this meant if the company wanted to follow up on this encouraging result, a new study would have to be started since the type 1 error of 0.05 had already been used up in the negative Phase 3 trial. This seemed like a waste of the money that was put into this study and more important of the contributions of the patients who participated. Intuitively, it seems that as you collect more information you should be able to become more certain about your conclusion without having to throw away everything you have learned up to a certain point. This experience prompted me to start thinking about the concepts of evidence we use in evaluating clinical trials.

Author

Eric Holmgren, Ph.D., received his B.S. in mathematics from the University of Nebraska in 1981. After receiving this degree he studied economics and finance for 2 years and then went on to Stanford University (California) where he received a Ph.D. in mathematical statistics in 1989. Once he graduated from Stanford, he went to work at Hoechst Roussel Pharmaceuticals in Bridgewater, New Jersey, where he worked on drugs for infections, diabetes, and HIV infection. He returned to the San Francisco Bay area in 1995 to work at Genentech as a senior statistician and later as a principal statistical scientist. While at Genentech, Dr. Holmgren worked on tPA for stroke, Avastin for colorectal cancer, and Herceptin for the adjuvant treatment of breast cancer. In 2010, he left Genentech to write this book and work as a consultant.

Introduction

Over the past 50 years, the discovery of new drugs that alleviate human suffering from diseases has been remarkable. From advances in treating and preventing heart disease to cures for some types of cancer, the impact on the lives of individuals in total is enormous. The financial resources that are employed in developing drugs are enormous as well. According to DiMasi et al. (2003), it takes close to $1 billion (2000 dollars) to develop a drug from its discovery in the lab to the point where physicians can use it to treat patients. Between the discovery of a molecule and its use by physicians to treat patients lies the enterprise of drug development. Drug development is the process by which drug companies test new molecules and assemble the necessary evidence required by regulatory agencies to show that a drug is safe and effective.

The development of a new drug requires input from many diverse areas such as biochemistry, biology, pharmacology, animal toxicology, medical science, and biostatistics. However, in its essence drug development is a collection of activities whereby a large pool of candidate molecules, most of which will not be successful, are tested in successive screening evaluations to determine which ones are more likely to be successful and will be further screened and ultimately evaluated in a Phase 3 clinical trial. The criteria for screening these molecules can be, for example, the results of *in vitro* cellular–based screening assays that are designed to detect properties that have the potential to provide the clinical benefit that is hoped for, results in animal models of the disease, or preliminary results in patients from small Phase 1 and Phase 2 trials. The establishment of the definitive evidence that the drug provides clinical benefit is accomplished by conducting a Phase 3 clinical trial.

The scientific rationale behind developing a particular drug to treat a specific disease typically involves manipulating a biologic target that has not been modified before. Although scientists may be able to describe how the drug modifies the target in their experiments and what changes may result on the cellular level, they cannot predict how a patient with the disease will respond to the new treatment. This is demonstrated by the relatively low rate of success of new molecules in Phase 3 trials, which is typically less than 50 percent among drugs that enter Phase 1 testing. So, while science can be used to select a good candidate molecule to be studied in clinical trials, it cannot be used to reliably ascertain which drug will be successful and which will not. That is, the scientific understanding of how a drug works cannot substitute for the results of a Phase 3 clinical trial.

The aim of this book is to quantify the basic elements of the clinical drug development process starting from Phase 1 clinical trials, consider its optimization under various circumstances, and evaluate the effectiveness of current approaches. The book looks at drug development not only from the perspective of a drug company but also from the perspective of a regulatory agency concerned about the quality of the drugs that are approved to be marketed. We start by briefly describing the clinical drug development process and providing an example.

Reference

DiMasi, J.A., Hansen, R.W., Grabowski, H.G. 2003. The price of innovation: New estimates of drug development costs. *J Health Economics* 22:151–185.

Section I

A Theory of Evaluating Drugs

1

Clinical Drug Development
Phases 1 through 3

The clinical development of new drugs traditionally takes place in three phases, starting with small studies that evaluate a handful of patients under carefully controlled conditions and ending with studies that enroll hundreds and sometimes even thousands of patients to develop the evidence necessary to achieve regulatory approval to market the new molecule. We start this chapter by briefly describing the three stages of clinical development and then give an example from the clinical area of oncology.

1.1 Stages of Clinical Development

In the first phase of clinical drug development the goal is to identify the maximum tolerable dose (MTD), which is the highest dose of the study drug that is deemed tolerable for most subjects. The MTD is usually determined in a small study where successive cohorts of only a handful of subjects receive progressively higher doses of the study drug as long as the previous dose was tolerable. Once a dose that is not tolerable has been identified, the next lowest dose that was studied is called the MTD. If the drug ultimately will be administered to patients for a long period of time, a Phase 1 single-dose MTD trial may be followed by a multiple-dose MTD trial.

In the second phase of drug development, the study drug's activity related to its potential clinical benefit is evaluated across a range of factors that may modify the magnitude of the treatment effect. These factors could include the dose of the study drug, the expression of a biomarker, or the type of disease. In some situations the study drug's activity can be evaluated in Phase 2 with a fully powered study on an efficacy endpoint that will support marketing approval. In most cases, however, the drug's activity has to be explored either with approvable endpoints in an underpowered trial or in fully powered trials with markers of activity that cannot support marketing approval.

If the activity of the study drug looks promising in Phase 2, then the drug enters the third phase of development where definitive evidence of clinical benefit is developed for regulatory authorities. In addition to developing evidence of clinical benefit, Phase 3 is used to develop evidence that the drug is safe enough to administer to the much wider population of patients that will receive it once marketing approval is granted.

1.2 Bevacizumab

To illustrate the three phases of drug development, the clinical development of the monoclonal antibody bevacizumab is presented. Bevacizumab was successfully developed as a treatment for colon cancer and thereafter as a treatment for a variety of other cancers such as lung and kidney. Figure 1.1 provides a description of the initial Phase 1 dose escalation trial for bevacizumab reported by Gordon et al. (2001).

Escalating doses of 0.1 mg/kg up to 10 mg/kg were evaluated in cohorts of 3 to 6 subjects in this Phase 1 trial. This study included both single-dose and multiple-dose segments. The single- and multiple-dose aspects of Phase 1 studies were combined in this trial to speed up the initiation of Phase 2 trials. Each subject received one dose of bevacizumab and was observed for 28 days. If after 28 days it appeared the subject tolerated the single dose of bevacizumab, the subject received three more doses so that the multiple-dose pharmacokinetics could be studied. If a group of 3 or 6 subjects had tolerated the drug well following 3 weeks of bevacizumab, then the next

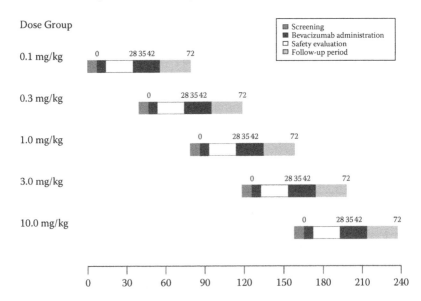

FIGURE 1.1
Study schema for a Phase 1 dose escalation trial.

higher dose was administered to a new cohort of subjects. Tolerating the drug meant that no more than 0 of 3 or 1 of 6 subjects experienced a dose-limiting toxicity. This study actually continued enrollment as planned up to the dose of 10 mg/kg and no dose-limiting toxicities were observed.

Following this Phase 1 dose escalation study there was a small study of bevacizumab in combination with chemotherapy to ensure that the combination was safe and tolerable (Margolin et al. 2001). A single dose of bevacizumab at a dose that was determined to be safe in the previous trial was studied with the standard chemotherapy regimens for colon, breast, and lung cancer. Three to six subjects were studied for each combination of bevacizumab with chemotherapy. Following completion of this combination Phase 1 trial, Phase 2 studies in larger number of subjects could be initiated without the concern that a large proportion of subjects enrolled in Phase 2 would be exposed to serious side effects of the drug.

The Phase 2 trial for bevacizumab in metastatic colon cancer was a randomized controlled trial that compared two doses of bevacizumab in combination with standard chemotherapy relative to standard chemotherapy alone in 104 subjects (Kabbinavar et al. 2003). The primary endpoints for the study were best confirmed response and time to progression. These two endpoints were not endpoints that could lead to marketing approval and moreover the study was not powered to detect the minimum clinically meaningful differences in these endpoints. Survival, which was the approvable endpoint in metastatic colon cancer at the time, was a secondary endpoint. The efficacy results for this Phase 2 trial are presented in Table 1.1.

TABLE 1.1

Phase 2 Efficacy Results

	Control ($N = 36$)	5 mg/kg ($N = 35$)	10 mg/kg ($N = 33$)
Confirmed Response			
Rate	17%	40%	24%
p-value (χ^2)		0.03	0.43
Time to Progression			
Median (months)	5.2	9.0	7.2
Hazard ratio		0.44	0.69
p-value (log-rank)		0.005	0.217
Survival Time			
Median (months)	13.8	21.5	16.1
Hazard ratio		0.63	1.17
p-value (log-rank)		0.137	0.582

Source: Adapted from Kabbinavar, F., Hurwitz, H., et al., 2003, Phase II, randomized trial comparing bevacizumab plus fluorouracil (FU)/leucovorin (LV) with FU/LV alone in patients with metastatic colorectal cancer, *J Clin Oncol* 21:60–65.

As can be seen in Table 1.1, the confirmed response rate was significantly better in the 5 mg/kg arm than in the control arm, and the 10 mg/kg arm was not better than the control. Time to progression in the 5 mg/kg arm was also significantly better than in the control arm, and in the 10 mg/kg arm it was not. Finally, in the case of survival there is a statistical "trend" favoring the 5 mg group over the control. With around 35 patients in the 5 mg and control arms, only a very strong survival benefit would be detectable at the 0.05 two-sided level of significance.

The results from this Phase 2 trial were sufficiently strong to prompt the initiation of a Phase 3 trial in colon cancer (Hurwitz et al. 2004). The two main arms of this Phase 3 trial enrolled more than 800 subjects. The survival results are presented in Table 1.2.

The Phase 3 study generated 399 events to evaluate the effect of bevacizumab on survival. These 399 events result in more than 80 percent power to detect a hazard ratio of 0.75, which is much better than the power to detect a survival benefit in the Phase 2 trial. As can be seen in Table 1.2, the result of the Phase 3 trial was highly statistically significant demonstrating that bevacizumab plus standard chemotherapy provided a survival benefit over standard chemotherapy alone. This evidence in favor of a treatment effect along with the safety information developed in the Phase 3 trial was sufficiently strong that the U.S. Food and Drug Administration granted marketing approval.

The clinical development of bevacizumab in colon cancer illustrates that a recurring issue in the drug development process is the question of how to properly size a study and then, once the data is collected and analyzed, how to decide whether to take the molecule to the next phase of development. The most important of these decisions is the decision to initiate Phase 3 trials following completion of Phase 2. As shown in Table 1.3 from Holmgren (2008), which is adapted from DiMasi et al. (2003), the average capitalized costs of Phase 3 trials are 4 times the costs of Phase 1 and 3 times the costs of Phase 2. Thus, it is not surprising that drug companies are much more contemplative

TABLE 1.2

Survival: Phase 3

	b-IFL + Placebo ($N = 411$)	b-IFL + AVF ($N = 402$)
Number of deaths	225	174
Percent surviving	45.3%	56.7%
Survival Time		
Median (months)	15.61	20.34
Hazard ratio		0.660
p-value (log-rank)		<0.0001

Source: Adapted from Hurwitz, H., Fehrenbacher, L., et al., 2004, Bevacizumab plus irinotecan, fluorouracil, and leucovorin for metastatic colorectal cancer, *N Engl J Med* 350:2335–2342.

about taking a molecule to Phase 3 than they are when taking a molecule into Phase 1 or Phase 2. We will start the study of the decision to move a molecule to the next phase of development with the study of the decision to move a molecule from Phase 2 to Phase 3. We will begin this analysis by considering the problems that arise when a drug company determines the size of the Phase 2 study and the decision criteria to initiate Phase 3 in such a way that shareholder value is "maximized."

References

DiMasi, J.A., Hansen, R.W., Grabowski, H.G. 2003. The price of innovation: New estimates of drug development costs. *J Health Economics* 22:151–185.

Gordon, M.S., Margolin, K., et al. 2001. Phase I safety and pharmacokinetic study of recombinant human anti-vascular endothelial growth factor in patients with advanced cancer. *J Clin Oncol* 19(3):843–850.

Holmgren, E.B. 2008. Are Phase 2 screening trials in oncology obsolete? *Stat Med* 27(4):556–567.

Hurwitz, H., Fehrenbacher, L., et al. 2004. Bevacizumab plus irinotecan, fluorouracil, and leucovorin for metastatic colorectal cancer. *N Engl J Med* 350:2335–2342.

Kabbinavar, F., Hurwitz, H., et al. 2003. Phase II, randomized trial comparing bevacizumab plus fluorouracil (FU)/leucovorin (LV) with FU/LV alone in patients with metastatic colorectal cancer. *J Clin Oncol* 21:60–65.

Margolin, K., Gordon, M.S., et al. 2001. Phase Ib trial of intravenous recombinant humanized monoclonal antibody to vascular endothelial growth factor in combination with chemotherapy in patients with advanced cancer: Pharmacologic and long-term safety data. *J Clin Oncol* 19(3):851–856.

2

Choosing Drugs to Develop

Most drug development takes place within a business enterprise where the objective is to maximize the value of the company's stock. Conceptually, the value of a company's stock is simply the present value of its expected future cash flows. That is

$$\text{Value of a company's stock} = \sum_{t=1}^{\infty} \frac{E(C_t)}{(1+r)^t} \qquad (2.1)$$

where C_t is the net cash flow generated by the company from all projects in year t, and r represents the discount rate used to determine the present value of a dollar earned one year in the future

The calculation of the expected future cash flow for a particular project in year t, $E(C_{\text{Project k in year }t})$, is accomplished in practice by splitting it into two components. Specifically

$$E(C_{\text{Project k in year }t}) = P(\text{Tech. Success}) \cdot E(C_{\text{Project k in year }t}/\text{Tech. Success}) \quad (2.2)$$

That is, the expected cash flow for project k in year t is the probability that the drug will be successfully developed multiplied by the expected cash flow in year t given that development was successful. The term $P(\text{Technical Success})$ is often referred to as PTS, which is short for probability of technical success.

The value of a company's stock can also be represented in terms of the value of individual projects as follows

$$\sum_{t=1}^{\infty} \frac{E(C_t)}{(1+r)^t} = \sum_{t=1}^{\infty} \frac{\sum_{k=1}^{\text{Projects}} E\left(C_{\text{Project k, year }t}\right)}{(1+r)^t} \qquad (2.3)$$

$$= \sum_{k=1}^{\text{Projects}} \sum_{t=1}^{\infty} \frac{E\left(C_{\text{Project k, year }t}\right)}{(1+r)^t} \qquad (2.4)$$

$$= \sum_{k=1}^{\text{Projects}} \sum_{t=1}^{\infty} \frac{P\left(\text{Tech. Success Proj k}\right) \cdot E\left(C_{\text{Project k, year }t} \mid \text{Tech. Success}\right)}{(1+r)^t} \quad (2.5)$$

$$= \sum_{k=1}^{\text{Projects}} P(\text{Tech. Success Project k}) \cdot \sum_{t=1}^{\infty} \frac{E\left(C_{\text{Project k, year t}} \mid \text{Tech. Success}\right)}{(1+r)^{t}} \quad (2.6)$$

That is, the value of a company's stock can be thought of as the weighted average of the expected discounted value of its drug projects where the weight is the PTS of each project. Projects that were successful will have a PTS of 1 while projects that failed will have a PTS of 0. Projects that are still in development will have a PTS between 0 and 1.

Although maximizing the value of a company's stock is conceptually straightforward, the details of determining the company's value can cause one to ponder whether such an approach indeed maximizes the value of the business. The specific details we consider here are the determination of PTS, the uncertainty in the expected future cash flows, and the question of whether the value of the business should be maximized today or in the future. The implications of these three issues will be discussed in the remainder of this chapter.

2.1 Probability of Technical Success

As long as the PTS for a project represents the probability that the project will be successful in that it equals the proportion of similar projects that would result in a positive Phase 3 trial, then the value of the company's stock can be represented as

$$\sum_{k=1}^{\text{Projects}} P(\text{Tech. Success Proj k}) \cdot \sum_{t=1}^{\infty} \frac{E\left(C_{\text{Project k, year t}} \mid \text{Tech. Success}\right)}{(1+r)^{t}} \quad (2.7)$$

$$= \sum_{k=1}^{\text{Projects}} E(I_{\{\text{Tech. Success Proj k}\}}) \cdot \sum_{t=1}^{\infty} \frac{E\left(C_{\text{Project k, year t}} \mid \text{Tech. Success Proj K}\right)}{(1+r)^{t}} \quad (2.8)$$

$$= E\left(\sum_{k=1}^{\text{Projects}} \sum_{t=1}^{\infty} \frac{I_{\{\text{Tech. Success Proj k}\}} \cdot C_{\text{Project k, year t}}}{(1+r)^{t}}\right) \quad (2.9)$$

To compute the value of the business on an empirical basis thus relies on the law of large numbers to estimate PTS as described in Equation (2.10)

$$\frac{1}{N} \sum_{j=1}^{N} I_{\{\text{Tech. Success Project k}\}} \rightarrow E\left(I_{\{\text{Tech. Success Project k}\}}\right) = P\left(\text{Tech. Success Project k}\right)$$

$$(2.10)$$

That is, if we could observe repeated independent trials of project k, then by the law of large numbers the proportion of those projects that are successful would approximate PTS and we could describe the variability of this estimate and a range of values that are likely to include the true PTS. Unfortunately, we can only observe the outcome of project k once and that is only after the project is complete. Indeed, the determination of PTS for a specific molecule cannot rely on the law of large numbers and empirical observation and can only represent the judgment of an individual or a group of individuals as to whether the molecule will be successful. Hence, the value of the company determined this way does not represent the discounted value of expected future cash flows in an empirical sense.

The absence of an empirical basis for determining the PTS for a specific molecule can be addressed by instead determining the PTS for classes of molecules and then assigning the PTS to a specific molecule based on which class it falls into. In other words, one could classify molecules according to important predictors of success, that is, is there another molecule with proven efficacy that hits the same target, the type of research (e.g., oncology, cardiovascular, diabetes), the research group that discovered the molecule, and so on, and estimate the probability of technical success for each class of molecules based on the outcomes of previous molecules that belong to each class. For example, Berkrot (2011) reported on a study by Eisenberg et al. that looked at success rates of drugs in various clinical areas. It was found that the highest success rates for moving from Phase 1 to approval were in infectious diseases such as hepatitis and HIV at 12 percent followed by diabetes at 10.4 percent and autoimmune diseases at 9.4 percent. The disease categories with the lowest success rates were cancer with a rate of 4.7 percent and cardiovascular with a rate of 5.7 percent. Grouping results of previous drug development projects according to such characteristics and potentially others would permit one to empirically calculate for each group the frequency with which it is successful and thereby assign an empirically based PTS to a new molecule.

If PTS is determined in this way and the success rates for classes of molecules are stable over time, then the value of the business calculated as in Equation (2.6) will be the discounted value of empirically based expected future cash flows. However, a key feature of drug development is the application of new techniques and the use of scientific discoveries to identify new drug candidates. Thus, the use of past frequencies of success may not always predict future success rates. It is interesting in this regard to note that Eisenberg found that the rate of success for drugs moving from Phase 1 to approval from the U.S. Food and Drug Administration (FDA) was about 1 in 10. This compares with rates of 1 in 5 and 1 in 6 that have been reported in earlier time periods. So at least at first glance it does not appear that the rates of success have been increasing over time.

2.2 Uncertainty Surrounding Expected Future Cash Flows

Another issue that raises doubt about the usefulness of making drug development decisions in a way that maximizes present value is the uncertainty surrounding expected future cash flows. Before a drug has received marketing approval, it is very hard to know how much cash it will generate because the strength of the treatment effect as well as the safety profile are unknown. To illustrate the consequences of this uncertainty suppose that a drug company has two types of projects to invest in. The present value of expected future cash flows are respectively PV_1 and PV_2 with associated required investments of Cost_1 and Cost_2. If we let k_1 and k_2 represent the number of projects of type 1 and 2 that are initiated, and we let B represent the budget that is available, then the strategy that maximizes the discounted value of expected future cash flows can be determined by maximizing the following objective function:

$$L = k_1 \cdot PV_1 + k_2 \cdot PV_2 + \lambda \cdot (k_1 \cdot \text{Cost}_1 + k_2 \cdot \text{Cost}_2 - B) \qquad (2.11)$$

Maximizing this objective function with respect to k_i, $\alpha_{2,i}, f_{N,i}$, and λ results in a maximization of $k_1 \cdot PV_1 + k_2 \cdot PV_2$ subject to the constraint that

$$k_1 \cdot \text{Cost}_1 + k_2 \cdot \text{Cost}_2 = B \qquad (2.12)$$

Taking partial derivatives with respect to k_i, $\alpha_{2,i}$, and $f_{N,i}$, leads to the following set of equations, which must be satisfied at the maximum. Here we have two thresholds, $\alpha_{2,i}$ for decision making in Phase 2 and two sample sizes for Phase 2, $f_{N,i}$, to allow for differences in the design and rules for decision making for projects with different present values for their cash flows. If we consider each type of project individually then the following equations must hold at the maximum.

$$\frac{\partial L}{\partial k_i} = PV_i + \lambda \cdot \text{Cost}_i = 0 \qquad (2.13)$$

$$\frac{\partial L}{\partial \alpha_{2,i}} = k_i \cdot \frac{\partial PV_i}{\partial \alpha_{2,i}} + \lambda \cdot k_i \cdot \frac{\partial \text{Cost}_i}{\partial \alpha_{2,i}} = 0 \qquad (2.14)$$

$$\frac{\partial L}{\partial f_{N,i}} = k_i \cdot \frac{\partial PV_i}{\partial f_{N,i}} + \lambda \cdot k_i \cdot \frac{\partial \text{Cost}_i}{\partial f_{N,i}} = 0 \qquad (2.15)$$

Equations (2.13) through (2.15) imply that the ratio, PV/Cost, is maximized with respect to $\alpha_{2,i}$ and $f_{N,i}$ since they imply that Equations (2.18) and (2.19), which are necessary conditions for maximizing PV/Cost, are also satisfied.

$$\frac{\partial PV_i/Cost_i}{\partial \alpha_{2,i}} = \frac{Cost_i \cdot \partial PV_i/\partial \alpha_{2,i} - PV_i \cdot \partial Cost_i/\partial \alpha_{2,i}}{Cost_i^2} = 0 \quad (2.16)$$

$$\frac{\partial PV_i/\partial \alpha_{2,i}}{Cost_i} - \frac{PV_i}{Cost_i} \cdot \frac{\partial Cost_i/\partial \alpha_{2,i}}{Cost_i} = 0 \quad (2.17)$$

$$\frac{\partial PV_i/\partial \alpha_{2,i}}{\partial Cost_i/\partial \alpha_{2,i}} = \frac{PV_i}{Cost_i} \quad (2.18)$$

and similarly for $\dfrac{\partial PV_i/Cost_i}{\partial f_N}$

$$\frac{\partial PV_i/\partial f_N}{\partial Cost_i/\partial f_N} = \frac{PV_i}{Cost_i} \quad (2.19)$$

Note that this ratio, PV/Cost, is proportional to efficiency, where the constant of proportionality does not depend on $\alpha_{2,i}$ and $f_{N,i}$. Thus, maximizing PV/Cost with respect to $\alpha_{2,i}$ and $f_{N,i}$ is the same as maximizing efficiency. We will introduce the concept of efficiency in Chapter 3.

We get a different answer to the optimization problem when considering the two types of projects together, in which case the optimal strategy is clearly to spend as much as possible on the projects with the highest ratio of *PV/Cost*. Indeed, if $PV_2/Cost_2 > PV_1/Cost_1$ and projects of type 2 are available, then the solution must be $k_2 = B/Cost_2$ and $k_1 = 0$.

Now if the company has spent as much as it could on project 2 but still has not exhausted the budget B, then the optimization problem the company faces is the same as earlier except that k_2 is fixed. In this situation, maximization is attained when

$$\frac{\partial L}{\partial k_1} = PV_1 + \lambda \cdot Cost_1 = 0 \quad (2.20)$$

$$\frac{\partial L}{\partial \alpha_{2,1}} = k_1 \cdot \frac{\partial PV_1}{\partial \alpha_{2,1}} + \lambda \cdot k_1 \cdot \frac{\partial Cost_1}{\partial \alpha_{2,1}} = 0 \quad (2.21)$$

$$\frac{\partial L}{\partial f_{N,1}} = k_1 \cdot \frac{\partial PV_1}{\partial f_{N,1}} + \lambda \cdot k_1 \cdot \frac{\partial Cost_1}{\partial f_{N,1}} = 0 \quad (2.22)$$

$$\frac{\partial L}{\partial \alpha_{2,2}} = k_2 \cdot \frac{\partial PV_2}{\partial \alpha_{2,2}} + \lambda \cdot k_2 \cdot \frac{\partial Cost_2}{\partial \alpha_{2,2}} = 0 \quad (2.23)$$

$$\frac{\partial L}{\partial f_{N,2}} = k_2 \cdot \frac{\partial PV_2}{\partial f_{N,2}} + \lambda \cdot k_2 \cdot \frac{\partial Cost_2}{\partial f_{N,2}} = 0 \quad (2.24)$$

The first three equations imply that the ratio, *PV/Cost*, for project 1 is maximized, whereas the last two equations imply that the ratio of the marginal change in *PV* to the marginal change in cost for project 2 when changing either α_2 or f_N is the same as the marginal change in *PV* to the marginal change in cost for project 1, which is the same as the ratio of *PV* to cost for project 1, (*K·Efficiency*).

Now we can show that maximizing present value as described earlier when there is uncertainty regarding the magnitude of the present value of returns if the drugs are successful does not come without costs. If there is in fact no difference between two drugs in terms of the magnitude of the present value of the returns but a company attempts to maximize its value based on estimated cash flows, the efficiency of drug development will be suboptimal and *a fortiori* net present value (NPV) will not be optimized either. The greater the uncertainty in the estimates of returns for each project, the greater the potential reduction in NPV due to a reduction in efficiency from following a strategy that attempts to maximize net present value.

The following example provides an illustration of the costs associated with maximizing present value when there is uncertainty surrounding the magnitude of the cash flows. In the example it is assumed that the cost functions are the same for the two projects and that the *PV* functions differ by a constant ($K = PV_2/PV_1$). Figure 2.1 displays the result of maximizing PV_2 subject to the constraints that

$$\frac{\partial PV_2/\partial \alpha_{2,2}}{\partial Cost/\partial \alpha_{2,2}} > \frac{PV_1}{Cost_1} \tag{2.25}$$

$$\frac{\partial PV_2/\partial f_{N,2}}{\partial Cost/\partial f_{N,2}} > \frac{PV_1}{Cost_1} \tag{2.26}$$

Note that as the estimated ratio PV_2/PV_1 increases the efficiency declines and that α_2 and f_N both increase, making it more likely that the Phase 3 trial will be started. In this example, the loss of efficiency (defined in the next chapter), from maximizing *PV* when the ratio of PV_2/PV_1 is more than 3 is $(0.125 - 0.10)/0.125 = 0.20$ or a decline of 20 percent. This observation raises the question whether it is worthwhile to chase what may or may not be greater cash flows when designing a Phase 2 trial if the cost may be a 20 percent reduction in the rate at which active drugs are discovered. It is hard to argue against maximizing PV in the drug development process until one realizes that there are costs associated with basing decisions on unreliable information.

It is interesting to note in the aforementioned example that simply maximizing efficiency for each project without regard to cash flow will maximize the minimum NPV when considering the returns on projects. This is true since maximizing efficiency when there is no difference between the two options maximizes NPV and this is where the minimum NPV is achieved.

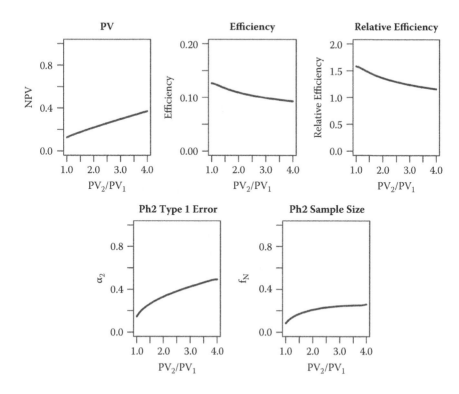

FIGURE 2.1
Impact of maximizing present value of cash flows on $\alpha_2, f_N,$ and efficiency.

2.3 Maximize the Value of the Company Today or Tomorrow?

Up to this point we have assumed that a business should maximize the value of its stock by maximizing the present value of expected future cash flows. Now we evaluate the present value framework itself as to whether it is appropriate for guiding decision making in the drug development process.

The impact of high expected returns on drug development decisions for a particular molecule is to reduce the minimum PTS required to go to the next stage of development regardless of the variability in those returns and the uncertainty in the estimates. This is a consequence of how capital markets value expected future returns, which is described by the capital asset pricing model of Sharpe (1964). In the capital asset pricing model, the variance of a stock's returns do not affect its value because the returns of an individual stock in a diversified stock portfolio are averaged with the returns of other stocks and hence the uncorrelated variability can be made as small as desired. Only the variability that is correlated with the return on the "market" affects the value of a company. In considering the value of a drug project, whether a particular drug is successful is not correlated with the general ups and downs of the economy, so this variability is ignored when valuing the company.

Drug stocks for small biotech or pharmaceutical companies have underlying cash flows that are highly skewed when compared with most other companies. If a drug succeeds there can be a large increase in the earnings, although the probability of success is often much less than 50 percent. This skewness in the distribution of cash flows for a biotech or pharmaceutical company can lead to a divergence over several drug projects between the expected return and the most likely return. The following example illustrates the discrepancy that can emerge between the expected and the most likely return.

Suppose that a new biotech company is considering a strategy to grow cash flows in the future. The strategy is to start with developing drugs for orphan indications where the clinical development costs are not too great. Following each success and as the cash flow for the company increases, the company will develop drugs with larger patient populations and larger clinical development costs. Two different kinds of drugs can be developed using this strategy. We will call these two types of drugs "Innovative" and "Me too." The returns from investing in the Innovative drug are

$$R_{Innovative} = \begin{cases} 2.4 \text{ with probability } 0.20 \\ 0.9 \text{ with probability } 0.80 \end{cases} \tag{2.27}$$

and the returns from investing in the Me too drug are

$$R_{Me\ too} = \begin{cases} 1.5 \text{ with probability } 0.40 \\ 0.9 \text{ with probability } 0.60 \end{cases} \tag{2.28}$$

Note that a return of 1 represents no gain and no loss on the investment.

The expected return for the Innovative drug type is 1.20, which is greater than the expected return of 1.14 for the Me too type, but it is riskier as well with a probability of success of just 20 percent. We also assume that the investment required for both drug types is the same, so in order to maximize net present value the Innovative drug type should be developed.

By the law of large numbers, the annual return on a portfolio of a large number of biotech companies using this strategy with Innovative drugs will be close to the expected return, 20 percent, assuming the outcome of drug projects for each company are independent. However, the most likely return over a period of T years is not 20 percent per year. The reason for this is seen in Equations (2.29) and (2.30). By the independence of drug projects the expected return will be

$$\left(E\left[\prod_{t=1}^{T} R_t\right]\right)^{1/T} = \left(\prod_{t=1}^{T} E[R_t]\right)^{1/T} = E[R_t] \qquad (2.29)$$

However, the geometric average return for an individual company over a period of T years converges as $T \to \infty$ to

$$\left[\prod_{t=1}^{T} R_t\right]^{1/T} = \exp\left(\frac{1}{T}\sum_{t=1}^{T}\log(R_t)\right) \to \exp\left(E\left[\log(R_t)\right]\right) = \exp(0.0908) = 1.095 \qquad (2.30)$$

by the law of large numbers on the log returns. Alternatively, we can write

$$\left[\prod_{t=1}^{T} R_t\right]^{1/T} = \exp\left(\frac{1}{T}\sum_{t=1}^{T}\log(R_t)\right) = \exp\left(\frac{1}{T}\sum_{t=1}^{T}E\left[\log(R_t)\right] + \frac{1}{T}\sum_{t=1}^{T}\varepsilon_t\right) \qquad (2.31)$$

where if $\text{var}(\varepsilon_t) < B$ for all t, then

$$\frac{1}{T}\sum_{t=1}^{T}\varepsilon_t \to_p 0 \qquad (2.32)$$

Now since the expected return is 20 percent per year and the annualized return converges to 9.5 percent per year, the probability of many of the outcomes in the sum that makes up the expected value, $\left(E\left[\prod_{t=1}^{T} R_{\text{Innovative}}^t\right]\right)^{1/T}$, must converge to zero as T gets large. This is illustrated in Figure 2.2.

Figure 2.2 is a graph of the returns for the Innovative and Me too strategies for growing the cash flows of a small biotech company over a course of 15 development projects. The figure graphs the cumulative probability of the number of successes versus the cumulative contribution to the expected return where the points are ordered from left to right by the number of successes. The expected number of successes in 15 drug projects is 3 for the Innovative strategy and 6 for the Me too strategy. Note that the cumulative probability ranges from 0 to 1, while the cumulative contribution to the expected value ranges from 0 to 15.4 = 1.2^{15} for the Innovative drug type and 0 to 7.14 = 1.14^{15} for the Me too drug type. Figure 2.2 shows that for the Innovative strategy, a little more than half of the expected return results from outcomes that in total have less than a 10 percent chance of occurring. Thus, 90 percent of the time the returns from the Innovative strategy will look similar to the returns from the Me too strategy.

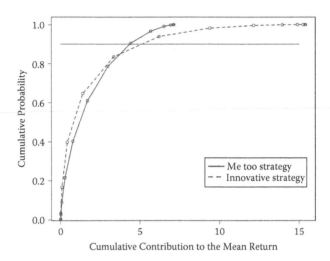

FIGURE 2.2
Probability of success versus the contribution to the expected return.

TABLE 2.1

Expected versus Most Likely Returns for
the Innovative and Me Too Strategies

Strategy	E(Return)	exp(E(log Return))
Innovative	1.20	1.095
Me too	1.14	1.104

The strategy that maximizes the most likely return in this example is the Me too strategy. The expected returns and the most likely returns for these two strategies are presented in Table 2.1.

Thus, maximizing expected returns instead of expected log returns will not necessarily optimize the most likely outcome in the future. Although the divergence in this particular example may seem small, the divergence between the expected outcome and the most likely outcome gets worse with a longer sequence of drug projects.

Is the divergence between the expected return and the most likely return less of an issue in a portfolio of similar companies? To address this question, Table 2.2 compares the cumulative probability of results from a 50-drug project strategy with the cumulative expected return of a portfolio of 1000 such companies. The probability that a single company using this strategy will see 20 or more successes out of 50 drug candidates is 0.001, yet the contribution of 20 or more successes to the expected value is 5037 of the 9100 total expected value. This is much worse than in the previous example where we considered a sequence of 15 drug projects. Now the probability of seeing one company with at least 25 successes in 50 attempts in a portfolio of

TABLE 2.2

Probability of Success versus the Contribution to the Expected Return: 50 Drug Projects in a Portfolio of 1000 Companies

					Property of Portfolio
	Properties of Individual Companies				Probability of Observing ≥
Number of Successes	Prob	Contribution to $E(R)$	Cum Prob	Cum Contribution to $E(R)$	Number of Successes in at Least One Company in a Portfolio of 1000 Companies
50	0.000	0.000	0.000	0.000	0.000
45	0.000	0.000	0.000	0.000	0.000
40	0.000	0.000	0.000	0.000	0.000
35	0.000	0.114	0.000	0.156	0.000
30	0.000	18.079	0.000	30.581	0.000
25	0.000	368.237	0.000	890.090	0.002
20	0.001	1042.533	0.001	5037.307	0.607
15	0.030	378.093	0.061	8609.424	1.000
10	0.140	13.103	0.556	9093.546	1.000
5	0.030	0.021	0.982	9100.434	1.000
0	0.000	0.000	1.000	9100.438	1.000

1000 companies is 0.002 and the contribution of at least 25 successes to the expected return of an individual company over 50 attempts is 890 out of 9100, almost 10 percent. So, even in a portfolio of 1000 companies, it is unlikely to see 25 or more successes in any of the companies, and so the return of the portfolio over this period of time will in most instances be close to 10 percent below the expected value. Although it is much better than for the company individually, the large number of stocks in a portfolio does not ensure that the expected return will be achieved.

Now let's consider how rebalancing can affect the returns of such a portfolio of stocks. It turns out that the 20 percent return on an annualized basis can be achieved if the portfolio is rebalanced after the completion of each drug project, with each company having the same weight as all the others after rebalancing. This is illustrated in Figure 2.3. The figure presents the results of a simulation that illustrates the benefit of rebalancing a portfolio of small biotech stocks after the completion of every drug project. We simulated the performance of two portfolios comprised of 1000 drug companies developing Innovative drugs over 50 successive periods. The first portfolio is rebalanced every year and the second one is not. The simulations include 1000 replications.

The simulations show that a portfolio where rebalancing is employed leads to returns over the 50 periods very tightly distributed around 1.20. On the other hand, the portfolio that is not rebalanced results in a distribution of returns that is highly skewed, with the mode of the distribution less than the expected return of 1.20.

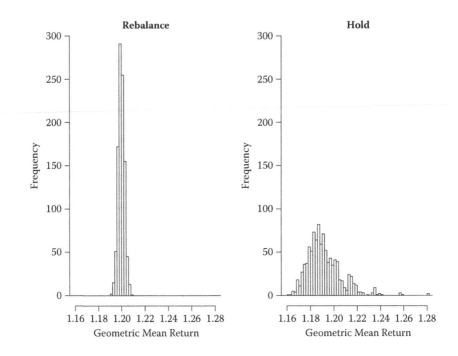

FIGURE 2.3
Rebalancing versus holding a portfolio of drug stocks.

Unfortunately, there is no mechanism whereby a company can rebalance itself. Thus, a company can either maximize NPV, which will maximize the value of the company today, or maximize the expected log returns, which will maximize the most likely value of the company in the future. If the company wishes to maximize its most likely value in the future, then it will maximize the expected log return, which gives less weight to the expected cash flows. This moves the decision-making criteria for the company from the maximization of NPV in the direction of maximizing efficiency, which is discussed in the next chapter.

Our simple example of a small biotech choosing a strategy to grow its cash flows differs from the real world in several respects. The most important of these is the fact that as a drug company grows, at some point it will start to invest in multiple projects to grow its cash flows, not a single one that gets larger and larger as the company grows. This has the effect of reducing the variability of the company's returns. And as the variability of the returns gets smaller, maximizing the expected log return will look more like maximizing the expected return. To see this, note that by Taylor's theorem

$$\log(r) = \log(E(R)) + \frac{1}{E(r)} \cdot (r - E(r)) - \frac{1}{E(r)^2} \cdot \frac{(r - E(r))^2}{2!} + R \qquad (2.33)$$

and so

$$E\big(\log(r)\big) - \log(E(R)) = -\frac{1}{E(r)^2} \cdot \frac{E\big(r - E(r)\big)^2}{2!} + R \to 0 \text{ as } \mathrm{var}(r) \to 0 \quad (2.34)$$

So, if strategy A for growing a company involves returns with a higher expected log return than for strategy B, eventually the actual realized return for strategy A will be greater than the actual realized return for strategy B. However, as noted earlier, as a company gets bigger it has to rely on multiple projects being successful each year for its growth, which reduces the variability of returns and pushes us back toward the situation where maximizing log returns is the same as maximizing returns.

2.4 Decision Rules for Phase 2

Putting aside the concerns laid out in this chapter regarding the use of PTS and the present value of future cash flows to guide drug development decision making, let's assume that we can determine PTS in a manner that will represent the frequency of successful development and that expected future cash flows can be known with some precision. Once a decision has been made to develop a new molecule based on the PTS of the molecule, data collected from Phase 2 studies could be used to update the probability of technical success and to determine whether Phase 3 studies should be initiated. More specifically, the data collected in Phase 2 could be used to construct a posterior probability of technical success using the initial estimate of PTS as a prior. The present value of expected cash flows could then be recalculated and gauged against the investment required to undertake Phase 3 and other investment options to determine whether further developing the drug would be consistent with maximizing the value of the company.

To be precise, let θ denote the treatment effect and suppose that θ_1 represents a treatment effect size consistent with technical success and θ_0 represents a treatment effect size consistent with no effect. Suppose that *PTS* represents the initial assessment that the drug will succeed, $P(\theta = \theta_1) = PTS$, and $f(x/\theta)$ represents the distribution of possible results from Phase 2, x, given θ. Then the posterior probability of technical success given x is

$$PTS_x = \frac{f(x/\theta_1) \cdot PTS}{f(x/\theta_1) \cdot PTS + f(x/\theta_0) \cdot (1 - PTS)} \quad (2.35)$$

If PTS_x times the present value of future cash flows is sufficiently great relative to the required investments, then development of the drug should proceed. If not, then development should cease. Now note that if f is a normal distribution, then

$$PTS_x = \frac{\exp\left(-\frac{1}{2}\left(\frac{x-\theta_1}{\sigma}\right)^2\right) \cdot PTS}{\exp\left(-\frac{1}{2}\left(\frac{x-\theta_1}{\sigma}\right)^2\right) \cdot PTS + \exp\left(-\frac{1}{2}\left(\frac{x-\theta_0}{\sigma}\right)^2\right) \cdot (1-PTS)} \qquad (2.36)$$

$$= \frac{1}{1+\exp\left(\frac{1}{2}\left(\frac{x-\theta_1}{\sigma}\right)^2 - \frac{1}{2}\left(\frac{x-\theta_0}{\sigma}\right)^2\right) \cdot \frac{(1-PTS)}{PTS}} \qquad (2.37)$$

and since

$$\frac{d}{dx}\left[\left(\frac{x-\theta_1}{\sigma}\right)^2 - \left(\frac{x-\theta_0}{\sigma}\right)^2\right] = \frac{1}{\sigma^2}\left(2 \cdot (x-\theta_1) - 2(x-\theta_0)\right) = \frac{2}{\sigma^2} \cdot (\theta_0 - \theta_1) \quad (2.38)$$

which is less than zero for $\theta_1 > \theta_0$, we have that PTS_x increases monotonically as x increases under those circumstances. On the other hand, if $\theta_1 < \theta_0$, we have that PTS_x increases monotonically as x decreases. Thus, a decision rule that requires NPV(x), as updated to reflect the Phase 2 results, to exceed some threshold is essentially the same as a decision rule that requires the observed data in Phase 2 or equivalently the associated Z-test exceed some threshold that is a function of the present value of the cash flows. The greater the present value of the cash flows, the lower the threshold for starting Phase 3.

Even though the aforementioned development relies on the ability to determine PTS as well as the ability to determine the present value of cash flows in the event of technical success, one could still construct decision rules of the form $x > B$ in the absence of any knowledge about PTS and the present value of future cash flows and evaluate their properties. The decision rules that we evaluate in the chapters that follow will all be of the form $x > B$. In essence, we will explore what are good choices for B.

2.5 Summary

In this chapter we described several deficiencies that stem from making drug development decisions that aim to maximize net present value. We noted that PTS, which is an essential element in the calculation of NPV, cannot be empirically based for an individual molecule and hence only represents the opinions of a group of individuals with regard to whether the drug will be successful. However, we pointed out that by determining PTS for classes of molecules instead of specific molecules, an NPV that does represent the discounted value of empirically based expected future cash flows can be determined. We showed that maximizing NPV for a new molecule can lead to a substantial reduction in the efficiency of identifying an active drug and hence that maximizing NPV where there is considerable uncertainty in future cash flows could ultimately reduce NPV. We showed that for small biotech or pharmaceutical companies with skewed cash flow distributions, maximizing $E(logR)$ will more likely lead to a company with greater value in the future than which would be attained when maximizing $E(R)$. Maximizing $E(logR)$ instead of $E(R)$ has the impact that bigger differences in the returns generated by different projects are required to alter the optimal Phase 2 design away from that which simply maximizes efficiency. And finally we showed even if one desired to maximize NPV in spite of these concerns, that the parameters of a Phase 2 trial that maximize the efficiency of drug development provide an important benchmark in determining the Phase 2 study design that maximizes NPV.

In Chapters 3 through 8, we develop a theory of drug development that is based on maximizing the efficiency with which drugs that truly provide clinical benefit are identified. That is, we consider how to optimize the drug development process so that the number of molecules that result in a positive Phase 3 trial per investment is maximized. Given the uncertainty in the cash flows that may result from the successful development of a new molecule, maximizing the number of successful molecules per investment as opposed to NPV per investment may be a reasonable strategy in most cases that a company may have to consider. In any event, understanding how to maximize the efficiency of drug development is necessary for ultimately maximizing NPV as well. After developing the theory of how to maximize the efficiency of drug development in the next several chapters, we turn to developing a theory of evidence for drug development. However, in Chapter 17 we return to the question of how to optimize drug development and present an example of how to maximize NPV per investment using the framework developed herein.

References

Berkrot, B. 2011. Success rate for experimental drugs falls: Study. https://www. p4healthcare.com/go/oncology/pbis/news.aspx?NewsItemId=20110214drgd003. xml (accessed August 8, 2012).

Sharpe, W.F. 1964. Capital asset prices: A theory of market equilibrium under conditions of risk. *J Finance* 19(3):425–442.

3

Phase 2/3 Strategy

In this chapter we describe how the decision-making criteria for determining whether to advance a molecule from Phase 2 to Phase 3 as well as the size of the Phase 2 study impacts the efficiency of drug development. To do this we specify a simple model of drug discovery and use it to evaluate the properties of Phase 2 studies and their associated decision rules.

3.1 Model

We start this assessment of the efficiency of drug development by modeling the drug discovery process as follows. Suppose that for any new molecule there are two possible states of nature. In one state of nature, the molecule has a clinical benefit relative to control that is represented by a treatment effect size of $\delta < 0$. In the second state of nature, the molecule is no different than control, which corresponds to a treatment effect of 0. We will let p represent the probability that the magnitude of the treatment effect is δ and will assume that p is greater than zero. This model views drug discovery as a process, where a certain proportion, p, of drug candidates that undergo clinical evaluation actually could provide clinical benefit to patients.

Let's adopt the following notation to describe the Phase 2 and Phase 3 studies. Let α_2 be the one-sided alpha level for Phase 2 testing, α_3 the one-sided alpha level for Phase 3 testing, and N the size of the Phase 3 trial. Further, let f_δ represent the magnitude of the treatment effect, $\delta = \left(\mu_T - \mu_C\right)/\sqrt{\sigma_T^2 + \sigma_C^2}$, in terms of the fraction of the treatment effect size used for planning Phase 3 and f_N represent the Phase 2 sample size as a fraction of the Phase 3 sample size. Finally, let β represent the power of the Phase 3 trial.

The family of all possible Phase 2 studies and associated decision rules can be written as $\{(\alpha_2, f_N)|0 \leq \alpha_2 \leq 1, f_N \geq 0\}$. Further, a number of important quantities can be written as presented in Table 3.1.

Recall that in Chapter 2 we noted that efficiency is proportional to PV/Cost. Given the expected cash flows, PV is proportional to P(Tech Success) and Cost is proportional to the expected number of subjects enrolled. Taking into account these relationships we can define the efficiency of drug development as

TABLE 3.1

Representations for Some Important Quantities in Phase 2/3 Studies

Power in Phase 3	$\Phi\left(z_{\alpha_3} - \left[z_{\alpha_3} - z_{\beta}\right] \cdot f_{\delta}\right)$
Power for Phase 3 endpoint in Phase 2	$\Phi\left(z_{\alpha_3} - \left[z_{\alpha_3} - z_{\beta}\right] \cdot f_{\delta} \cdot \sqrt{f_N}\right)$
Probability of a positive Phase 3 due to an active drug	$p \cdot \Phi\left(z_{\alpha_3} - \left[z_{\alpha_3} - z_{\beta}\right] \cdot f_{\delta} \cdot \sqrt{f_N}\right) \cdot \Phi\left(z_{\alpha_3} - \left[z_{\alpha_3} - z_{\beta}\right] \cdot f_{\delta}\right)$
Expected number of subjects enrolled in Phase 2 and Phase 3	$N \cdot \left[f_N + p \cdot \Phi\left(z_{\alpha_2} - \left[z_{\alpha_3} - z_{\beta}\right] \cdot f_{\delta} \cdot \sqrt{f_N}\right) + (1-p) \cdot \alpha_2\right]$

$$\text{Efficiency} = \frac{\text{P(Technical Success)}}{\text{E(Number of Subjects Enrolled)}} \quad (3.1)$$

Here we take the probability of technical success to be determined as described in Chapter 2 for a class of molecules rather than for a specific molecule. Using the expressions for these quantities in Table 3.1, the efficiency of a Phase 2/3 clinical trial program can then be formally defined as

$$\frac{p \cdot \Phi\left(z_{\alpha_2} - \left[z_{\alpha_3} - z_{\beta}\right] \cdot f_{\delta} \cdot \sqrt{f_N}\right) \cdot \Phi\left(z_{\alpha_3} - \left[z_{\alpha_3} - z_{\beta}\right] \cdot f_{\delta}\right)}{N \cdot \left[f_N + p \cdot \Phi\left(z_{\alpha_2} - \left[z_{\alpha_3} - z_{\beta}\right] \cdot f_{\delta} \cdot \sqrt{f_N}\right) + (1-p) \cdot \alpha_2\right]} \quad (3.2)$$

In essence, efficiency can be viewed as the rate per expected number of subjects enrolled in Phase 2 and Phase 3 trials at which a clinical development strategy identifies active drugs with a positive Phase 3 trial. The greater the efficiency, the greater the number of drugs with clinical benefit that are identified per subjects enrolled in Phase 2/3 clinical trial programs.

Appendix A will show that maximizing the efficiency as defined earlier is the same as maximizing the expected number of successful Phase 3 studies due to active drugs subject to a constraint on the number of subjects enrolled. Note that the probability of a positive Phase 3 trial when there is no clinical benefit is not included in the numerator of the expression for efficiency. This outcome is not considered technical success because drugs that are approved and do not have a "true" benefit may end up creating obligations for the company that more than offset any potential revenue.

Figure 3.1 and Figure 3.2 illustrate how the principal parts of efficiency, namely, the probability of a positive Phase 3 trial due to an active drug and the expected sample size in Phase 2/3, change as the Phase 2 trial changes, that is, as α_2 (the type 1 error with which testing is carried out in Phase 2) and f_N (the fraction of the number of subjects enrolled in Phase 3 that are actually enrolled in Phase 2) change. In addition, the figures examine how the efficiency of a Phase 2/3 program changes as a result of these changes in its components.

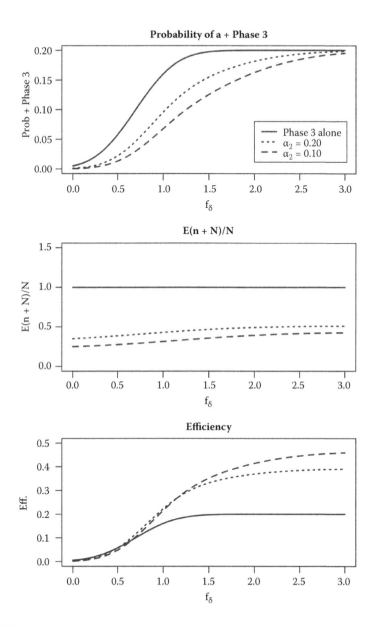

FIGURE 3.1
Properties of a clinical development program with a Phase 2 trial preceding Phase 3. $p = 0.2$, $f_N = 0.15$.

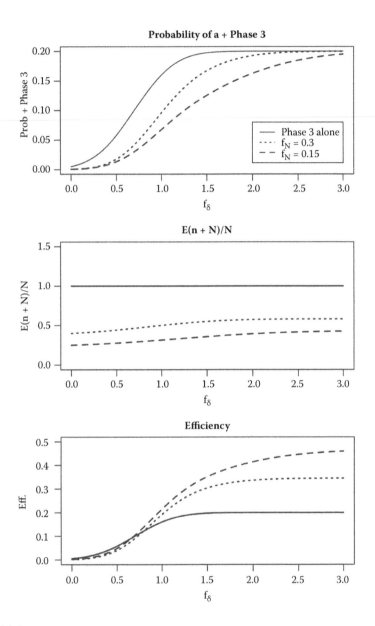

FIGURE 3.2
Properties of a clinical development program with a Phase 2 trial preceding Phase 3. $p = 0.2$, $\alpha_2 = 0.1$.

The solid lines in the figures represent a simple Phase 2/3 development program consisting only of a Phase 3 study with 80 percent power at the planned treatment effect size ($f_\delta = 1$). The dotted lines in Figure 3.1 represent the same Phase 3 study accompanied by a Phase 2 study with $f_N = 0.15$ and $\alpha_2 = 0.1$ or $\alpha_2 = 0.2$ one sided, and the dotted lines in Figure 3.2 denote an accompanying Phase 2 study with $f_N = 0.15$ or $f_N = 0.30$ and $\alpha_2 = 0.1$ one sided. p, the probability that the drug is active, is taken to be 0.20 in Figure 3.1 and Figure 3.2.

The figures show that reducing either α_2 or f_N decreases the probability of a positive Phase 3 trial and the expected enrollment. The third panel in the figures illustrate that decreasing α_2 increases the efficiency for $f_\delta > 1.0$, whereas decreasing f_N increases the efficiency for $f_\delta > 0.8$.

It is easy to see why as either α_2 or f_N decreases, the probability of a positive Phase 3 and the expected number of subjects should decrease. This follows since as α_2 or f_N decreases, it is harder to start a Phase 3.

It is more difficult to see the impact of reducing α_2 or f_N on efficiency. But this can be inferred by noting that the limit of efficiency as f_δ gets large is

$$\lim_{f_\delta \to +\infty} \frac{p \cdot \Phi\left(z_{\alpha_2} - \left[z_{\alpha_3} - z_\beta\right] \cdot f_\delta \cdot \sqrt{f_N}\right) \cdot \Phi\left(z_{\alpha_3} - \left[z_{\alpha_3} - z_\beta\right] \cdot f_\delta\right)}{N \cdot \left[f_N + p \cdot \Phi\left(z_{\alpha_2} - \left[z_{\alpha_3} - z_\beta\right] \cdot f_\delta \cdot \sqrt{f_N}\right) + (1-p) \cdot \alpha_2\right]}$$

$$= \frac{p}{N[f_N + p + (1-p)\alpha_2]} \tag{3.3}$$

So for large treatment effects, reducing either α_2 or f_N increases the efficiency.

3.2 When Is a Phase 2/3 Strategy Better Than a Phase 3 Trial Alone?

This section addresses the question: When is a Phase 2/3 strategy better than a Phase 3 trial alone? The first step toward answering this question is rewriting the efficiency of a Phase 2/3 development program as follows

$$Eff_{ClinDev} = \frac{p \cdot \Phi\left(z_{\alpha_3} - \left[z_{\alpha_3} - z_\beta\right] \cdot f_\delta\right)}{N} \cdot \frac{\Phi\left(z_{\alpha_2} - \left[z_{\alpha_3} - z_\beta\right] \cdot f_\delta \cdot \sqrt{f_N}\right)}{p \cdot \Phi\left(z_{\alpha_2} - \left[z_{\alpha_3} - z_\beta\right] \cdot f_\delta \cdot \sqrt{f_N}\right) + (1-p) \cdot \alpha_2 + f_N} \tag{3.4}$$

The term on the left represents the efficiency of a clinical development program consisting only of a Phase 3 trial. The term on the right, which we will call the relative efficiency, thus represents the efficiency of a Phase 2/3 program relative to the efficiency of a single Phase 3 study. That is, the relative efficiency is the factor by which the efficiency of a clinical development program consisting only of a Phase 3 trial changes by preceding the definitive Phase 3 trial with a Phase 2 screening study. If the relative efficiency is greater than 1 then the Phase 2 trial increases the efficiency of clinical development while if the relative efficiency is less than one it decreases the efficiency.

Efficiency as quantified above represents the number of approvals per expected number of subjects enrolled in Phase 2 and Phase 3 trials. By changing the expression for efficiency slightly the question of how Phase 2 helps or hinders the whole drug development process can be addressed. The key to this change is to incorporate the cost of drug development prior to Phase 2 into the denominator.

If we represent the pre-Phase 2 drug development costs with the variable C, then the efficiency of a whole drug development program can be expressed as

$$\frac{p \cdot \Phi\left(z_{\alpha_2}-\left[z_{\alpha_3}-z_\beta\right] \cdot f_\delta \cdot \sqrt{f_N}\right) \cdot \Phi\left(z_{\alpha_2}-\left[z_{\alpha_3}-z_\beta\right] \cdot f_\delta\right)}{C+N\cdot\left[f_N+p\cdot\Phi\left(z_{\alpha_2}-\left[z_{\alpha_3}-z_\beta\right]\cdot f_\delta\cdot\sqrt{f_N}\right)+(1-p)\cdot\alpha_2\right]} \tag{3.5}$$

Note that the costs represented by C are in units of subjects enrolled in order that they may be added to the expected enrollment in Phase 2 and Phase 3. Now we can express the efficiency for the whole drug development process as

$Efficiency_{DrugDevelopment}$

$$= \frac{p \cdot \Phi\left(z_{\alpha_3}-\left[z_{\alpha_3}-z_\beta\right]\cdot f_\delta\right)}{C+N}$$

$$\times \frac{\Phi\left(z_{\alpha_2}-\left[z_{\alpha_3}-z_\beta\right]\cdot f_\delta\cdot\sqrt{f_N}\right)}{\left\{f_N+p\cdot\Phi\left(z_{\alpha_2}-\left[z_{\alpha_3}-z_\beta\right]\cdot f_\delta\cdot\sqrt{f_N}\right)+(1-p)\cdot\alpha_2+\dfrac{C}{N}\right\}\cdot\dfrac{N}{C+N}} \tag{3.6}$$

A Phase 2/3 design again provides a benefit in terms of the efficiency of drug development over a program without a Phase 2 trial if the second term in the product above is greater than 1, that is, if

$$\frac{\Phi\left(z_{\alpha_2}-\left[z_{\alpha_3}-z_\beta\right]\cdot f_\delta\cdot\sqrt{f_N}\right)}{\left\{f_N+p\cdot\Phi\left(z_{\alpha_2}-\left[z_{\alpha_3}-z_\beta\right]\cdot f_\delta\cdot\sqrt{f_N}\right)+(1-p)\cdot\alpha_2+\dfrac{C}{N}\right\}\cdot\dfrac{N}{C+N}} > 1 \tag{3.7}$$

Now the inequality in Equation (3.7) implies

$$\left\{p\cdot\Phi\left(z_{\alpha_2}-\left[z_{\alpha_3}-z_\beta\right]\cdot f_\delta\cdot\sqrt{f_N}\right)+(1-p)\cdot\alpha_2+f_N\right\}$$

$$< \Phi\left(z_{\alpha_2}-\left[z_{\alpha_3}-z_\beta\right]\cdot f_\delta\cdot\sqrt{f_N}\right)-\left\{1-\Phi\left(z_{\alpha_2}-\left[z_{\alpha_3}-z_\beta\right]\cdot f_\delta\cdot\sqrt{f_N}\right)\right\}\cdot\frac{C}{N} \tag{3.8}$$

and further rearranging terms produces

$$\frac{\Phi\left(z_{\alpha_2}-\left[z_{\alpha_3}-z_\beta\right]\cdot f_\delta\cdot\sqrt{f_N}\right)-\left\{1-\Phi\left(z_{\alpha_2}-\left[z_{\alpha_3}-z_\beta\right]\cdot f_\delta\cdot\sqrt{f_N}\right)\right\}\cdot\dfrac{C}{N}}{p\cdot\Phi\left(z_{\alpha_2}-\left[z_{\alpha_3}-z_\beta\right]\cdot f_\delta\cdot\sqrt{f_N}\right)+(1-p)\cdot\alpha_2+f_N}>1 \qquad (3.9)$$

This expression in Equation (3.9) mirrors the expression in Equation (3.4) for the relative efficiency of a Phase 2/3 clinical trial program where there are no discovery costs prior to Phase 2 to consider. Indeed, note that when $C = 0$, the second expression in the numerator of Equation (3.9) is zero and the expression as a whole reduces to the relative efficiency in Equation (3.4). The expression in Equation (3.9) shows that the impact of discovery costs on whether a Phase 2 trial is beneficial is to offset the power of the Phase 2 study by the type 2 error multiplied by the ratio of pre-Phase 2 costs to Phase 3 costs. Thus, the set of f_δ where a Phase 2 study improves the efficiency of drug development is reduced after accounting for discovery costs.

3.3 How Much Can Efficiency Be Improved?

The amount by which efficiency can be improved by a Phase 2 trial depends on the value of C, that is, the costs to develop a molecule to the point of initiating Phase 2 trials. If one is considering only the efficiency of a Phase 2/3 clinical trial program, then C is set equal to zero. C is also set equal to zero if one is considering the development of a new indication for an approved molecule. But what should C be when considering the development of a new molecule?

Of course the costs for each molecule will be different. And if one has at hand the development costs for the molecule as well as the estimated costs of Phase 3, then those numbers should be used. To give us a general idea of how pre-Phase 2 development costs compare to the costs of Phase 3 trials we refer to Holmgren (2008, Table 3), which breaks down the cost of developing a drug in the pharmaceutical industry into the preclinical and clinical phases based on DiMasi et al. (2003).

Before testing can begin on a molecule in a Phase 2 trial, substantial costs are incurred in Phase 1 testing as well as in testing that occurs prior to the first-in-man trial. The costs per molecule entering Phase 2 not only represent the costs incurred on direct testing of the molecule but also include the costs incurred for molecules that did not make it to the point of starting Phase 2. More precisely, we can say that the total costs incurred prior to the initiation of Phase 2 are the preclinical costs plus the Phase 1 costs per molecule, all divided by the probability that a single molecule will enter Phase 2. Using the capitalized cost data from DiMasi et al. (2003), we can estimate the pre-Phase 2 cost as $(72.0 + 30.5)/0.71 = \$144$ million (in 2000 dollars). If the Phase 2 trial is ultimately successful, then the cost of the follow-up Phase 3 trial will be $119.2 million. So we can conclude that the costs incurred prior to initiating Phase 2 are approximately equal to the costs of a Phase 3 trial.

Table 3.2 presents the relative efficiency of a Phase 2/3 development program across a range of several factors: the probability that the drug provides a clinical benefit, p; the magnitude of the treatment effect, f_δ; the discovery costs, C; the type 1 error in Phase 2; and the fraction of the Phase 3 sample size that is enrolled in the Phase 2 trial. Relative efficiencies greater than 1 are highlighted in the table. Recall that when the relative efficiency is greater than 1, the Phase 2 trial improves the efficiency of the drug development process as measured by the number of active molecules that are successful in Phase 3 per investment.

First, consider the case where the probability that the drug is active is 0.20. It can be seen from Table 3.2 that when $C = 0$ and the true treatment effect varies from 75 to 150 percent of what was planned for in Phase 3, the maximum improvement in efficiency ranges from 16 to 71 percent. On the other hand, when $C = 1$ the corresponding improvement in efficiency ranges from −6 to 12 percent.

Now note that as the probability that the drug is active decreases from 0.20 to 0.05, the efficiency increases. For example, when the probability that the drug is active in Table 3.2 is 0.05 and $C = 0$ the maximum improvement in efficiency ranges from 29 to 119 percent instead of 16 to 70 percent when $p = 0.20$. The improvement in efficiency when $p = 0.05$ and $C = 1$ is −4 to 19 percent, which compares to −6 to 12 percent when $p = 0.20$.

Regardless of the value of p, it can be seen that there is a big difference in the degree to which efficiency improves when $C = 1$ and $C = 0$, and hence that the magnitude of C needs to be taken into account when considering whether to undertake a Phase 2 screening trial. If developing a new molecule, it may not be wise to use a Phase 2 screening trial. Indeed, a Phase 2 screening trial with a small value for α_2 can substantially reduce the efficiency of drug development, whereas the best trial would only marginally improve efficiency by testing at a one-sided alpha level of 0.30 to 0.50, which is not very informative. The exception to this would be when the probability of an active drug is 0.05 and the objective is to find a treatment with an effect size 50 percent greater than what would be used to size the Phase 3 trial, specifically the minimum clinically meaningful difference. In this situation an appropriately designed Phase 2 trial can increase the efficiency by at least 19 percent. As noted in Chapter 2, drugs for clinical areas such as cancer and cardiovascular tend to have lower values for the probability of success, whereas drugs such as anti-infectives have higher rates of success.

If instead the development of a new indication for an approved molecule is under consideration, then utilizing a Phase 2 screening trial can improve the efficiency of development. An appropriately chosen α level for decision making in Phase 2 can result in an improvement in efficiency of 30 percent or more over a Phase 3 trial alone depending on the value for p.

TABLE 3.2

Relative Efficiency of a Phase 2/3 Development Program Compared to a Single Phase 3 Trial without a Preceding Phase 2

Probability Drug Is Active	C	β	f_δ	α_2	f_N 0.2	0.4	0.6	0.8	1
0.05	0	0.8	0.75	0.025	0.66	0.60	0.58	0.55	0.53
				0.050	0.93	0.81	0.73	0.68	0.63
				0.100	1.17	1.00	0.87	0.78	0.70
				0.200	1.29	1.10	0.95	0.82	0.73
				0.300	1.28	1.09	0.93	0.81	0.71
				0.400	1.22	1.04	0.89	0.77	0.68
				0.500	1.15	0.99	0.84	0.73	0.64
0.05	0	0.8	1.00	0.025	1.02	0.96	0.89	0.82	0.75
				0.050	1.31	1.16	1.03	0.91	0.80
				0.100	1.53	1.30	1.10	0.95	0.82
				0.200	1.56	1.31	1.09	0.92	0.79
				0.300	1.47	1.23	1.02	0.86	0.74
				0.400	1.35	1.13	0.95	0.80	0.70
				0.500	1.24	1.04	0.88	0.75	0.65
0.05	0	0.8	1.25	0.025	1.44	1.32	1.17	1.01	0.88
				0.050	1.73	1.48	1.24	1.04	0.88
				0.100	1.88	1.54	1.25	1.03	0.86
				0.200	1.79	1.44	1.16	0.95	0.80
				0.300	1.61	1.30	1.06	0.88	0.75
				0.400	1.45	1.18	0.96	0.81	0.70
				0.500	1.30	1.07	0.89	0.75	0.66
0.05	0	0.8	1.50	0.025	1.89	1.64	1.35	1.11	0.92
				0.050	2.14	1.72	1.36	1.10	0.91
				0.100	2.19	1.69	1.31	1.05	0.87
				0.200	1.97	1.51	1.18	0.96	0.81
				0.300	1.72	1.34	1.07	0.88	0.75
				0.400	1.51	1.20	0.97	0.81	0.70
				0.500	1.34	1.08	0.89	0.75	0.66
0.05	1	0.8	0.75	0.025	0.25	0.37	0.45	0.51	0.54
				0.050	0.38	0.51	0.59	0.63	0.65
				0.100	0.56	0.68	0.74	0.75	0.74
				0.200	0.76	0.85	0.86	0.84	0.80
				0.300	0.87	0.92	0.90	0.86	0.81
				0.400	0.93	0.94	0.90	0.85	0.80
				0.500	0.96	0.95	0.89	0.83	0.78
0.05	1	0.8	1.00	0.025	0.39	0.59	0.71	0.76	0.78
				0.050	0.55	0.75	0.83	0.85	0.84
				0.100	0.74	0.90	0.94	0.92	0.87

(Continued)

TABLE 3.2 (*Continued*)

Relative Efficiency of a Phase 2/3 Development Program Compared to a Single Phase 3 Trial without a Preceding Phase 2

Probability Drug Is Active	C	β	f_δ	α_2	f_N 0.2	0.4	0.6	0.8	1
				0.200	0.93	1.01	0.99	0.93	0.87
				0.300	1.01	1.03	0.98	0.92	0.85
				0.400	1.04	1.02	0.96	0.89	0.82
				0.500	1.04	1.00	0.93	0.86	0.79
0.05	1	0.8	1.25	0.025	0.56	0.83	0.93	0.94	0.91
				0.050	0.74	0.96	1.01	0.98	0.92
				0.100	0.92	1.07	1.06	1.00	0.92
				0.200	1.07	1.12	1.05	0.97	0.89
				0.300	1.11	1.10	1.02	0.93	0.86
				0.400	1.11	1.07	0.98	0.90	0.82
				0.500	1.09	1.03	0.94	0.86	0.79
0.05	1	0.8	1.50	0.025	0.75	1.04	1.08	1.03	0.95
				0.050	0.93	1.13	1.12	1.04	0.95
				0.100	1.09	1.19	1.12	1.02	0.93
				0.200	1.19	1.18	1.08	0.98	0.89
				0.300	1.19	1.13	1.03	0.94	0.86
				0.400	1.17	1.08	0.98	0.90	0.82
				0.500	1.13	1.03	0.94	0.86	0.79
0.1	0	0.8	0.75	0.025	0.65	0.59	0.56	0.54	0.52
				0.050	0.89	0.78	0.71	0.66	0.61
				0.100	1.12	0.96	0.84	0.75	0.68
				0.200	1.24	1.06	0.91	0.80	0.71
				0.500	1.13	0.97	0.83	0.72	0.63
0.1	0	0.8	1.00	0.025	0.97	0.91	0.86	0.79	0.73
				0.050	1.24	1.10	0.98	0.87	0.77
				0.100	1.44	1.23	1.05	0.91	0.79
				0.200	1.48	1.24	1.04	0.89	0.76
				0.500	1.21	1.02	0.86	0.74	0.64
0.1	0	0.8	1.25	0.025	1.35	1.24	1.11	0.97	0.84
				0.050	1.61	1.39	1.17	0.99	0.85
				0.100	1.74	1.44	1.18	0.98	0.83
				0.200	1.68	1.36	1.11	0.92	0.78
				0.500	1.27	1.04	0.87	0.74	0.65
0.1	0	0.8	1.50	0.025	1.74	1.52	1.27	1.05	0.88
				0.050	1.95	1.59	1.28	1.04	0.87
				0.100	2.00	1.57	1.24	1.00	0.84
				0.200	1.83	1.43	1.13	0.92	0.78
				0.500	1.30	1.05	0.87	0.74	0.65

TABLE 3.2 (*Continued*)

Relative Efficiency of a Phase 2/3 Development Program Compared to a Single Phase 3 Trial without a Preceding Phase 2

Probability Drug Is Active	C	β	f_δ	α_2	f_N				
					0.2	0.4	0.6	0.8	1
0.1	1	0.8	0.75	0.025	0.25	0.36	0.45	0.50	0.54
				0.050	0.38	0.51	0.58	0.62	0.64
				0.100	0.55	0.67	0.72	0.74	0.73
				0.200	0.75	0.83	0.84	0.82	0.79
				0.500	0.95	0.94	0.88	0.83	0.77
0.1	1	0.8	1.00	0.025	0.38	0.58	0.69	0.75	0.76
				0.050	0.54	0.73	0.82	0.84	0.82
				0.100	0.73	0.88	0.92	0.90	0.86
				0.200	0.91	0.99	0.97	0.92	0.86
				0.500	1.03	0.99	0.92	0.85	0.78
0.1	1	0.8	1.25	0.025	0.55	0.81	0.91	0.92	0.89
				0.050	0.73	0.94	0.99	0.96	0.90
				0.100	0.91	1.05	1.04	0.97	0.90
				0.200	1.05	1.10	1.03	0.95	0.87
				0.500	1.08	1.01	0.93	0.85	0.78
0.1	1	0.8	1.50	0.025	0.74	1.01	1.05	1.00	0.93
				0.050	0.91	1.10	1.09	1.01	0.93
				0.100	1.06	1.16	1.09	1.00	0.91
				0.200	1.16	1.15	1.06	0.96	0.88
				0.500	1.11	1.02	0.93	0.85	0.78
0.15	0	0.8	0.75	0.025	0.63	0.57	0.55	0.52	0.50
				0.050	0.86	0.75	0.69	0.64	0.59
				0.100	1.08	0.92	0.81	0.73	0.66
				0.200	1.20	1.02	0.88	0.77	0.69
				0.300	1.19	1.02	0.88	0.77	0.68
				0.400	1.15	0.99	0.85	0.74	0.65
				0.500	1.10	0.94	0.81	0.71	0.62
0.15	0	0.8	1.00	0.025	0.93	0.88	0.82	0.76	0.70
				0.050	1.18	1.05	0.94	0.84	0.75
				0.100	1.36	1.17	1.01	0.87	0.76
				0.200	1.41	1.19	1.00	0.86	0.74
				0.300	1.35	1.13	0.95	0.81	0.70
				0.400	1.26	1.06	0.90	0.77	0.67
				0.500	1.18	0.99	0.84	0.72	0.63
0.15	0	0.8	1.25	0.025	1.27	1.17	1.05	0.92	0.81
				0.050	1.50	1.30	1.11	0.95	0.82
				0.100	1.62	1.35	1.12	0.94	0.80
				0.200	1.58	1.29	1.06	0.88	0.75

(Continued)

TABLE 3.2 (*Continued*)

Relative Efficiency of a Phase 2/3 Development Program Compared to a Single Phase 3 Trial without a Preceding Phase 2

					f_N				
Probability Drug Is Active	C	β	$f_δ$	$α_2$	0.2	0.4	0.6	0.8	1
				0.300	1.46	1.20	0.98	0.83	0.71
				0.400	1.34	1.10	0.91	0.77	0.67
				0.500	1.23	1.01	0.85	0.73	0.63
0.15	0	0.8	1.50	0.025	1.61	1.42	1.19	1.00	0.84
				0.050	1.79	1.48	1.21	0.99	0.83
				0.100	1.84	1.47	1.17	0.96	0.81
				0.200	1.71	1.35	1.08	0.89	0.76
				0.300	1.54	1.23	0.99	0.83	0.71
				0.400	1.39	1.12	0.92	0.78	0.67
				0.500	1.26	1.02	0.85	0.73	0.63
0.15	1	0.8	0.75	0.025	0.25	0.36	0.44	0.49	0.53
				0.050	0.38	0.50	0.57	0.61	0.63
				0.100	0.55	0.66	0.71	0.73	0.72
				0.200	0.74	0.82	0.83	0.81	0.78
				0.300	0.85	0.89	0.87	0.83	0.79
				0.400	0.91	0.92	0.88	0.83	0.78
				0.500	0.94	0.93	0.88	0.82	0.76
0.15	1	0.8	1.00	0.025	0.38	0.57	0.68	0.73	0.75
				0.050	0.54	0.72	0.80	0.82	0.81
				0.100	0.72	0.87	0.90	0.88	0.84
				0.200	0.90	0.97	0.95	0.90	0.84
				0.300	0.98	1.00	0.95	0.89	0.82
				0.400	1.01	1.00	0.93	0.86	0.80
				0.500	1.02	0.98	0.91	0.84	0.77
0.15	1	0.8	1.25	0.025	0.54	0.79	0.89	0.90	0.87
				0.050	0.71	0.92	0.97	0.94	0.89
				0.100	0.89	1.03	1.01	0.95	0.88
				0.200	1.03	1.07	1.01	0.93	0.86
				0.300	1.08	1.06	0.98	0.90	0.83
				0.400	1.08	1.03	0.95	0.87	0.80
				0.500	1.07	1.00	0.92	0.84	0.78
0.15	1	0.8	1.50	0.025	0.72	0.99	1.03	0.98	0.91
				0.050	0.89	1.08	1.06	0.99	0.91
				0.100	1.04	1.13	1.07	0.98	0.89
				0.200	1.14	1.13	1.03	0.94	0.86
				0.300	1.15	1.09	0.99	0.91	0.83
				0.400	1.13	1.05	0.96	0.87	0.80
				0.500	1.10	1.01	0.92	0.84	0.78

TABLE 3.2 (*Continued*)

Relative Efficiency of a Phase 2/3 Development Program Compared to a Single Phase 3 Trial without a Preceding Phase 2

Probability Drug Is Active	C	β	f_δ	α_2	f_N				
					0.2	0.4	0.6	0.8	1
0.2	0	0.8	0.75	0.025	0.61	0.56	0.53	0.51	0.49
				0.050	0.83	0.73	0.67	0.62	0.58
				0.100	1.04	0.89	0.79	0.71	0.64
				0.200	1.15	0.99	0.86	0.75	0.67
				0.300	1.16	0.99	0.85	0.75	0.66
				0.400	1.12	0.96	0.83	0.72	0.64
				0.500	1.08	0.93	0.80	0.70	0.62
0.2	0	0.8	1.00	0.025	0.89	0.84	0.79	0.74	0.68
				0.050	1.12	1.00	0.90	0.80	0.72
				0.100	1.29	1.11	0.96	0.84	0.74
				0.200	1.34	1.14	0.96	0.83	0.72
				0.300	1.29	1.09	0.92	0.79	0.69
				0.400	1.22	1.03	0.87	0.75	0.65
				0.500	1.15	0.97	0.82	0.71	0.62
0.2	0	0.8	1.25	0.025	1.20	1.11	1.00	0.88	0.78
				0.050	1.40	1.23	1.06	0.91	0.78
				0.100	1.52	1.28	1.07	0.90	0.77
				0.200	1.49	1.23	1.02	0.85	0.73
				0.300	1.39	1.15	0.95	0.80	0.69
				0.400	1.29	1.07	0.89	0.76	0.66
				0.500	1.19	0.99	0.83	0.71	0.62
0.2	0	0.8	1.50	0.025	1.49	1.33	1.13	0.95	0.81
				0.050	1.65	1.39	1.14	0.95	0.80
				0.100	1.71	1.38	1.11	0.92	0.78
				0.200	1.60	1.28	1.04	0.86	0.74
				0.300	1.47	1.18	0.96	0.81	0.69
				0.400	1.34	1.08	0.89	0.76	0.66
				0.500	1.22	1.00	0.83	0.71	0.62
0.2	1	0.8	0.75	0.025	0.25	0.36	0.44	0.49	0.52
				0.050	0.37	0.50	0.57	0.61	0.62
				0.100	0.54	0.66	0.70	0.72	0.71
				0.200	0.73	0.81	0.82	0.80	0.77
				0.300	0.84	0.88	0.86	0.82	0.78
				0.400	0.90	0.91	0.87	0.82	0.77
				0.500	0.94	0.92	0.87	0.81	0.76
0.2	1	0.8	1.00	0.025	0.38	0.57	0.67	0.72	0.73
				0.050	0.53	0.71	0.79	0.80	0.79
				0.100	0.71	0.85	0.88	0.86	0.83

(*Continued*)

TABLE 3.2 (*Continued*)

Relative Efficiency of a Phase 2/3 Development Program Compared to a Single Phase 3 Trial without a Preceding Phase 2

Probability Drug Is Active	C	β	f_δ	α_2	f_N 0.2	0.4	0.6	0.8	1
				0.200	0.88	0.96	0.94	0.89	0.83
				0.300	0.96	0.98	0.94	0.87	0.81
				0.400	1.00	0.98	0.92	0.85	0.79
				0.500	1.01	0.97	0.90	0.83	0.77
0.2	1	0.8	1.25	0.025	0.54	0.78	0.87	0.88	0.85
				0.050	0.70	0.90	0.95	0.92	0.87
				0.100	0.87	1.00	0.99	0.93	0.87
				0.200	1.01	1.05	0.99	0.92	0.84
				0.300	1.06	1.04	0.97	0.89	0.82
				0.400	1.06	1.02	0.94	0.86	0.79
				0.500	1.05	0.99	0.91	0.83	0.77
0.2	1	0.8	1.50	0.025	0.71	0.96	1.00	0.96	0.89
				0.050	0.87	1.05	1.03	0.97	0.89
				0.100	1.02	1.10	1.04	0.96	0.88
				0.200	1.11	1.10	1.01	0.92	0.85
				0.300	1.12	1.07	0.98	0.89	0.82
				0.400	1.11	1.03	0.94	0.86	0.79
				0.500	1.08	1.00	0.91	0.83	0.77

There are several other things to note in Table 3.2. It will be observed that as the treatment effect increases, the relative efficiency increases as well. Indeed, this relationship between the treatment effect size and efficiency can be deduced from the derivative of the relative efficiency with respect to f_δ.

$$\frac{\partial \text{Rel Eff}}{\partial f_\delta}$$

$$= \frac{\left[(1-p)\cdot\alpha_2 + f_N + C/N\right]\cdot\phi\left(z_{\alpha_2}-\left[z_{\alpha_3}-z_\beta\right]\cdot f_\delta\cdot\sqrt{f_N}\right)\cdot(-1)\cdot(z_{\alpha_3}-z_\beta)\cdot\sqrt{f_N}}{\left(p\cdot\Phi\left(z_{\alpha_2}-\left[z_{\alpha_3}-z_\beta\right]\cdot f_\delta\cdot\sqrt{f_N}\right)+(1-p)\cdot\alpha_2 + f_N + C/N\right)^2\cdot N/(C+N)}$$

$$> 0 \hspace{4cm} (3.10)$$

This expression is positive since all terms are positive except (–1) and $(z_{\alpha_3}-z_\beta)$. When these two terms are combined the result is positive and thus the whole expression is positive. That is, the gain in efficiency afforded by a Phase 2 screening study increases as the treatment effect increases. And it increases up to

$$\lim_{f_\delta \to \infty} \text{Rel Eff} = \frac{1}{\{f_N + p + (1-p)\cdot\alpha_2 + C/N\}\cdot\dfrac{N}{C+N}} \qquad (3.11)$$

Next, note that as p, the probability of success, decreases, the relative efficiency increases. This follows since the derivative of the relative efficiency with respect to p is

$$\frac{\partial\text{Rel Eff}}{\partial p}$$

$$= \frac{\Phi\Big(z_{\alpha_2} - \big[z_{\alpha_3} - z_\beta\big]\cdot f_\delta\cdot\sqrt{f_N}\Big)\cdot(-1)\cdot\Big[\Phi\Big(z_{\alpha_2} - \big[z_{\alpha_3} - z_\beta\big]\cdot f_\delta\cdot\sqrt{f_N}\Big) - \alpha_2\Big]\cdot\dfrac{N}{C+N}}{\Big(\big[p\cdot\Phi\big(z_{\alpha_2} - \big[z_{\alpha_3} - z_\beta\big] < 0\cdot f_\delta\cdot\sqrt{f_N}\big) + (1-p)\cdot\alpha_2 + f_N + C/N\big]\dfrac{N}{C+N}\Big)^2}$$

$$< 0 \qquad (3.12)$$

which is less than zero since $\big[z_{\alpha_3} - z_\beta\big] < 0$. Thus, the relative efficiency increases as p decreases to zero and it increases to

$$\lim_{p\to 0} \text{Rel Eff} = \frac{\Phi\Big(z_{\alpha_2} - \big[z_{\alpha_3} - z_\beta\big]\cdot f_\delta\cdot\sqrt{f_N}\Big)}{\big(f_N + \alpha_2 + C/N\big)\cdot\dfrac{N}{C+N}} \qquad (3.13)$$

On the other hand, as p increases to 1, the relative efficiency decreases to

$$\lim_{p\to 1} \text{Rel Eff} = \frac{\Phi\Big(z_{\alpha_2} - \big[z_{\alpha_3} - z_\beta\big]\cdot f_\delta\cdot\sqrt{f_N}\Big)}{\Big(f_N + \Phi\big(z_{\alpha_2} - \big[z_{\alpha_3} - z_\beta\big]\cdot f_\delta\cdot\sqrt{f_N}\big) + C/N\Big)\cdot\dfrac{N}{C+N}} \qquad (3.14)$$

Now

$$\Phi\Big(z_{\alpha_2} - \big[z_{\alpha_3} - z_\beta\big]\cdot f_\delta\cdot\sqrt{f_N}\Big) = \Phi\Big(z_{\alpha_2} - \big[z_{\alpha_3} - z_\beta\big]\cdot f_\delta\cdot\sqrt{f_N}\Big)\cdot\frac{N}{C+N}$$

$$+ \Phi\Big(z_{\alpha_2} - \big[z_{\alpha_3} - z_\beta\big]\cdot f_\delta\cdot\sqrt{f_N}\Big)\cdot\frac{C}{C+N} \qquad (3.15)$$

$$< \Big[f_N + \Phi\Big(z_{\alpha_2} - \big[z_{\alpha_3} - z_\beta\big]\cdot f_\delta\cdot\sqrt{f_N}\Big)\Big]\cdot\frac{N}{C+N} + 1\cdot\frac{C}{C+N} \qquad (3.16)$$

$$= \Big[f_N + \Phi\Big(z_{\alpha_2} - \big[z_{\alpha_3} - z_\beta\big]\cdot f_\delta\cdot\sqrt{f_N}\Big) + \frac{C}{N}\Big]\cdot\frac{N}{C+N} \qquad (3.17)$$

and so the limit of the relative efficiency as $p \to 1$ is less than 1 regardless of the value of C. Thus, if the probability of technical success is very close to 1, the relative efficiency will be less than 1 and a Phase 2 clinical trial will not help improve the drug development process.

Figure 3.3 and Figure 3.4 present as a function of the treatment effect size, the maximum relative efficiency that can be achieved where the maximum is taken over the Phase 2 type 1 error, α_2, and sample size, f_N. They describe the most by which a Phase 2 trial could improve the efficiency of drug development if we knew the true treatment effect size, f_δ, in advance.

Figure 3.3 shows that if the pre-Phase 2 costs are close to zero, then there is some Phase 2 trial with α_2 less than one and f_N greater than zero that will result in a relative efficiency greater than one, that is, there exists a Phase 2 trial that will improve the drug development process compared with a Phase 3 trial alone. On the other hand, Figure 3.4 shows that if the pre-Phase 2 costs are approximately equal to the Phase 3 costs, as is the case for a new molecule, then there is a Phase 2 trial that will improve the efficiency of the drug development process as long as the treatment effect size is at least as large as what will be used in planning for Phase 3. If the treatment effect size is less, then the optimal Phase 2 trial is to not do one at all ($\alpha_2 = 1, f_N = 0$).

As already noted, Figures 3.3 and 3.4 show the most that efficiency can be improved as a function of f_δ. When we plan a Phase 2 study we do not know the magnitude of the drug's treatment effect, f_δ, and so cannot design the Phase 2 study to maximize the efficiency for detecting a particular drug as was done to produce Figure 3.3 and Figure 3.4. However, we should not set up a clinical program to optimize the detection of the treatment effect for a particular drug understudy, whatever the true treatment effect might be. Rather we should set up our clinical programs to optimize the discovery of drugs with treatment effects that we are interested in. The figures can help guide the design of the Phase 2 trial to optimize the discovery of drugs with treatment effects of interest.

3.4 Admissible Phase 2 Trial Designs

In this section, another approach is taken to aiding the design of the Phase 2 trial. Here we identify those Phase 2 study designs that cannot be uniformly improved upon by another. That is, we identify an admissible family of Phase 2 designs, a family of procedures where each member of the family is such that there does not exist another procedure with uniformly greater efficiency for all f_δ. Thus, when planning a Phase 2 study, the design should be selected from the admissible family by whatever criteria is relevant.

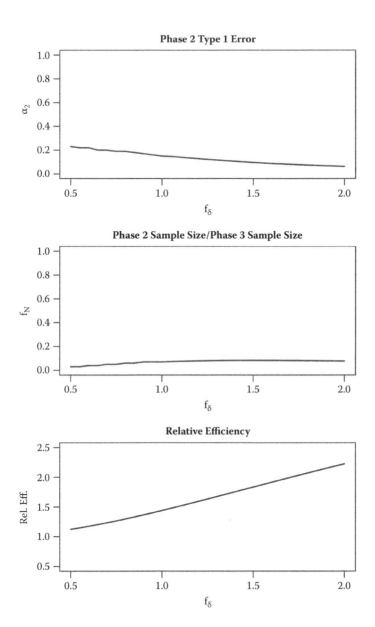

FIGURE 3.3
Phase 2 study parameters that maximize relative efficiency as a function of the treatment effect size. $C/N = 0$.

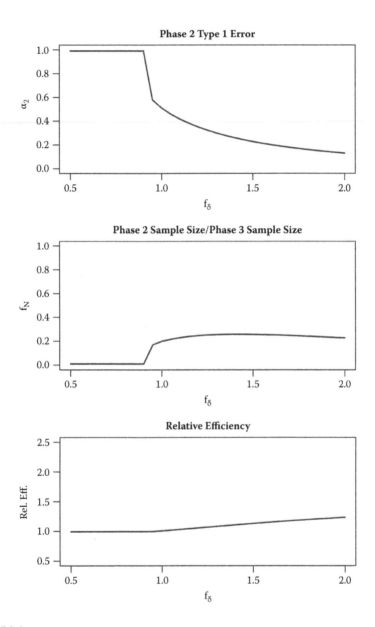

FIGURE 3.4
Phase 2 study parameters that maximize relative efficiency as a function of the treatment effect
size. $C/N = 1$.

As a first step toward determining an admissible family of Phase 2 designs, let's consider what limits on the Phase 2 trial can be deduced from simply requiring that the efficiency of the Phase 2/3 program must be better than the efficiency of a Phase 3 trial alone. The efficiency of a Phase 2/3 program is dominated or strictly inferior to the efficiency of just a single Phase 3 study with no Phase 2 component if the relative efficiency is less than 1 for all $f_\delta > 0$. Now since the relative efficiency increases monotonically as f_δ increases, the relative efficiency will be greater than 1 for some f_δ if and only if $\lim_{f_\delta \to \infty}$ Rel Eff > 1. Now note that $\lim_{f_\delta \to \infty}$ Rel Eff is

$$\lim_{f_\delta \to \infty} \frac{\Phi\left(z_{\alpha_2} - \left[z_{\alpha_3} - z_\beta\right] \cdot f_\delta \cdot \sqrt{f_N}\right)}{\left\{f_N + p \cdot \Phi\left(z_{\alpha_2} - \left[z_{\alpha_3} - z_\beta\right] \cdot f_\delta \cdot \sqrt{f_N}\right) + (1-p) \cdot \alpha_2 + \dfrac{C}{N}\right\} \cdot \dfrac{N}{C+N}} \tag{3.18}$$

$$= \frac{1}{\left\{f_N + p \cdot 1 + (1-p) \cdot \alpha_2 + \dfrac{C}{N}\right\} \cdot \dfrac{N}{C+N}} \tag{3.19}$$

Thus, if a Phase 2/Phase 3 clinical development program is not strictly inferior to a Phase 3 trial alone, that is, if it is admissible, it must satisfy

$$\frac{1}{\left\{f_N + p \cdot 1 + (1-p) \cdot \alpha_2 + \dfrac{C}{N}\right\} \cdot \dfrac{N}{C+N}} > 1 \tag{3.20}$$

which reduces to

$$(1 - [p + (1-p)\,\alpha_2]) \geq f_N \tag{3.21}$$

Note that as $p \to 1$ (the molecule under study is active with high probability) the inequality will not be satisfied, whereas as $p \to 0$ the inequality becomes $(1 - \alpha_2) \geq f_N$. Table 3.3 presents the resulting limits on a Phase 2 trial in terms of the ratio f_N for various values of p and α_2.

Phase 2/3 development programs that incorporate a Phase 2 trial with fewer subjects as a percentage of the Phase 3 sample size than is indicated in Table 3.3 are not completely inferior to a Phase 3 trial alone in the sense that there is a range of values for f_δ for which the relative efficiency is greater than 1. So for example, if a drug company has a track record where 20 percent of the drugs that enter Phase 2 are successful, then a Phase 2/3 development program that consists of a Phase 2 trial that tests for activity at α_2 one-sided equal to 0.20 followed by a Phase 3 trial will not be inferior in terms of efficiency to a Phase 3 trial alone for all f_δ if the sample size for the Phase 2 trial is less than or equal to 64 percent of the Phase 3 sample size.

Now we develop an admissible family of Phase 2 studies. We utilize a theorem of Wald (1947) to develop this family. Recall that relative efficiency is

TABLE 3.3

Limits on the Ratio of the Sample Size in Phase 2 to the Sample Size in Phase 3, f_N

Probability of an Active Drug	One-Sided Alpha Level for Phase 2 Testing						
	0.025	0.05	0.10	0.20	0.30	0.40	0.50
0.05	0.93	0.90	0.86	0.76	0.66	0.57	0.48
0.10	0.88	0.86	0.81	0.72	0.63	0.54	0.45
0.15	0.83	0.81	0.76	0.68	0.60	0.51	0.43
0.20	0.78	0.76	0.72	0.64	0.56	0.48	0.40
0.25	0.73	0.71	0.68	0.60	0.52	0.45	0.38
0.30	0.68	0.66	0.63	0.56	0.49	0.42	0.35
0.35	0.63	0.62	0.58	0.52	0.45	0.39	0.32
0.40	0.58	0.57	0.54	0.48	0.42	0.36	0.30
0.45	0.54	0.52	0.50	0.44	0.38	0.33	0.27
0.50	0.49	0.48	0.45	0.40	0.35	0.30	0.25

$$RE(\alpha_2, f_N, f_\delta) = \frac{\Phi\left(z_{\alpha_2} - \left[z_{\alpha_3} - z_\beta\right] \cdot f_\delta \cdot \sqrt{f_N}\right)}{\left\{p \cdot \Phi\left(z_{\alpha_2} - \left[z_{\alpha_3} - z_\beta\right] \cdot f_\delta \cdot \sqrt{f_N}\right) + (1-p) \cdot \alpha_2 + f_N + C/N\right\} \cdot N/(C+N)}$$

(3.22)

By Wald's theorem an essentially complete class of Phase 2 screening trials is comprised of all Phase 2 screening trials (α_2, f_N) that maximize

$$\int RE(\alpha_2, f_N, f_\delta) \cdot g(f_\delta) \cdot df_\delta \tag{3.23}$$

for some prior $g(f_\delta)$. So, the following two equations must be satisfied for some $g(f_\delta)$ if (α_2, f_N) is in the essentially complete class:

$$\frac{\partial}{\partial \alpha_2} \int RE(\alpha_2, f_N, f_\delta) \cdot g(f_\delta) \cdot df_\delta = 0 \tag{3.24}$$

$$\frac{\partial}{\partial f_N} \int RE(\alpha_2, f_N, f_\delta) \cdot g(f_\delta) \cdot df_\delta = 0 \tag{3.25}$$

Appendix B presents the derivation of an algorithm for determining this family of Phase 2 trials. Table 3.4 describes the resulting boundary for different values of C/N.

Table 3.4 provides a more restrictive upper limit on the size of a Phase 2 trial expressed as a fraction of the Phase 3 sample size than was provided in Table 3.3. This limit is calculated for a range of probabilities of developing an effective drug, p, a range of one-sided type 1 errors in Phase 2, α_2, and pre-Phase 2 development costs represented by $C/N = 0$, 0.5, and 1.0.

TABLE 3.4

Upper Limit on f_N to Ensure That a Phase 2 Screening Trial Is Admissible

p	α_2	Ratio of Pre-Phase 2 Costs to Phase 3 Costs		
		($C/N = 0$)	($C/N = 0.5$)	($C/N = 1.0$)
0.1	0.025	0.055	0.091	0.097
0.1	0.050	0.074	0.145	0.146
0.1	0.100	0.092	0.198	0.219
0.1	0.200	0.055	0.230	0.265
0.1	0.500	—	0.156	0.202
0.2	0.025	0.049	0.079	0.082
0.2	0.050	0.067	0.131	0.129
0.2	0.100	0.083	0.180	0.200
0.2	0.200	0.044	0.210	0.244
0.2	0.500	—	0.152	0.200
0.4	0.025	0.038	0.067	0.067
0.4	0.050	0.051	0.091	0.097
0.4	0.100	0.059	0.133	0.146
0.4	0.200	0.034	0.171	0.185
0.4	0.500	—	0.129	0.159

If a Phase 2 trial satisfies the limits on f_N presented in Table 3.4, then no other Phase 2 trial will have uniformly greater relative efficiency for all treatment effect sizes greater than 0. On the other hand, if f_N does not satisfy the constraint in Table 3.4, there will exist a Phase 2 study design with greater relative efficiency for all treatment effect sizes greater than zero.

From Table 3.4 we see that if a drug company has a track record where 20 percent of the drugs that enter Phase 2 are successful, then the efficiency of a clinical development plan for a new molecule ($C/N = 1.0$), which includes a Phase 2 trial that tests for activity at α_2 one-sided = 0.20 with a sample size greater than or equal to 24 percent of the Phase 3 sample size, can be uniformly improved upon for all f_δ greater than zero by another Phase 2 trial.

3.5 Projects That Are Not Least Attractive

In Chapter 2, the potential drawbacks of making drug development decisions in ways that maximize net present value (NPV) were pointed out. If after considering these points one still wishes to maximize NPV, then the following observations would apply.

If there exists a Phase 2 study that improves the efficiency of a clinical trial program for the project with the lowest PV/Cost ratio in the portfolio, then for each project in the portfolio there exists a Phase 2 trial that will improve the present value of the company's portfolio where the improvement goes to zero as the magnitude of the present value of the cash flow increases. To see this recall that the present value is proportional to

$$p \cdot \Phi\left(z_{\alpha_2} - \left[z_{\alpha_3} - z_\beta\right] \cdot f_\delta \cdot \sqrt{f_N}\right) \cdot \Phi\left(z_{\alpha_3} - \left[z_{\alpha_3} - z_\beta\right] \cdot f_\delta \cdot \sqrt{f_N}\right) \qquad (3.26)$$

and the cost is proportional to

$$C + N \cdot \left[f_N + p \cdot \Phi\left(z_{\alpha_2} - \left[z_{\alpha_3} - z_\beta\right] \cdot f_\delta \cdot \sqrt{f_N}\right) + (1-p) \cdot \alpha_2\right] \qquad (3.27)$$

Thus,

$$\frac{PV}{Cost} = K \cdot \frac{p \cdot \Phi\left(z_{\alpha_2} - \left[z_{\alpha_3} - z_\beta\right] \cdot f_\delta \cdot \sqrt{f_N}\right) \cdot \Phi\left(z_{\alpha_3} - \left[z_{\alpha_3} - z_\beta\right] \cdot f_\delta \cdot \sqrt{f_N}\right)}{C + N \cdot \left[f_N + p \cdot \Phi\left(z_{\alpha_2} - \left[z_{\alpha_3} - z_\beta\right] \cdot f_\delta \cdot \sqrt{f_N}\right) + (1-p) \cdot \alpha_2\right]} \qquad (3.28)$$

and

$$\frac{\partial PV / \partial \alpha_2}{\partial Cost / \partial \alpha_2} = K \cdot \frac{\dfrac{p}{N} \cdot \dfrac{\phi\left(z_{\alpha_2} - \left[z_{\alpha_3} - z_\beta\right] \cdot f_\delta \cdot \sqrt{f_N}\right)}{\phi(z_{\alpha_2})}}{p \cdot \dfrac{\phi\left(z_{\alpha_2} - \left[z_{\alpha_3} - z_\beta\right] \cdot f_\delta \cdot \sqrt{f_N}\right)}{\phi(z_{\alpha_2})} + (1-p)} \qquad (3.29)$$

Now note that

$$\frac{\phi\left(z_{\alpha_2} - \left[z_{\alpha_3} - z_\beta\right] \cdot f_\delta \cdot \sqrt{f_N}\right)}{\phi(z_{\alpha_2})} \qquad (3.30)$$

is monotone decreasing as a function of α_2 since

$$\frac{d}{dx} \frac{\phi(x+\delta)}{\phi(x)} = -\delta \cdot \frac{\phi(x+\delta)}{\phi(x)} < 0 \qquad (3.31)$$

for δ greater than zero. Further

$$\frac{\phi(x+\delta)}{\phi(x)} \qquad (3.32)$$

decreases to zero as x goes to infinity since

$$\frac{\phi(x+\delta)}{\phi(x)} \leq \frac{\phi(x+\delta)}{\dfrac{d}{dx}\phi(x+\delta) \cdot (-\delta) + \phi(x+\delta)} \qquad (3.33)$$

$$= \frac{\phi(x+\delta)}{(-1)\cdot(x+\delta)\cdot\phi(x+\delta)\cdot(-\delta)+\phi(x+\delta)} = \frac{1}{1+x\cdot\delta+\delta^2} \to 0 \qquad (3.34)$$

Thus, $\dfrac{\partial PV/\partial\alpha_2}{\partial Cost/\partial\alpha_2}$, as a function of α_2, is monotone, decreasing to zero. Now note that if a project has a higher $PV/Cost$ ratio than the least favorable project then the ratio $\dfrac{\partial PV/\partial\alpha_2}{\partial Cost/\partial\alpha_2}$ will be higher as well since the factor K in Equations (3.28) and (3.29) will be greater than it is for the lowest PV/Cost project. So we can conclude that the α_2 level for any project is greater than the α_2 level for the least PV/Cost project in order that the ratio $\dfrac{\partial PV/\partial\alpha_2}{\partial Cost/\partial\alpha_2}$ will be the same for all projects. Thus, if there does not exist a Phase 2 study that improves efficiency for the least PV/Cost project (that is, α_2 is equal to 1), then there does not exist a Phase 2 study for any project in the portfolio that will improve PV of the portfolio since α_2 for those projects must be 1 as well. Conversely, if there exists a Phase 2 trial that improves efficiency for the least PV/Cost project, then for each project in the portfolio there exists a Phase 2 trial that will improve the PV for the portfolio of projects. This is the case since the conditions for maximizing PV subject to the budget constraint are met for α_2 less than 1 and $f_N > 0$. That is, since

$$\frac{\partial PV_2/\partial\alpha_2}{\partial Cost_2/\partial\alpha_2}\left(\alpha_2^{1*}\right) > \frac{\partial PV_1/\partial\alpha_2}{\partial Cost_1/\partial\alpha_2}\left(\alpha_2^{1*}\right) = \frac{PV_1}{Cost_1} \qquad (3.35)$$

and

$$\lim_{\alpha_2\to1}\frac{\partial PV_2/\partial\alpha_2}{\partial Cost_2/\partial\alpha_2}\left(\alpha_2\right) = 0 \qquad (3.36)$$

by continuity there exists an α_2^{2*} such that

$$\frac{\partial PV_2/\partial\alpha_2}{\partial Cost_2/\partial\alpha_2}\left(\alpha_2^{2*}\right) = \frac{\partial PV_1/\partial\alpha_2}{\partial Cost_1/\partial\alpha_2}\left(\alpha_2^{1*}\right) = \frac{PV_1}{Cost_1} \qquad (3.37)$$

which is the condition that must be satisfied to maximize PV of the portfolio. As the difference in PV/Cost between the least value project and the project at hand increases, α_2 goes to one and f_N goes to zero. And as α_2 goes to one and f_N goes to zero, the efficiency of drug development will decline. In the extreme, maximizing PV will imply not doing a Phase 2 trial.

3.6 Example: Bevacizumab

In this section we evaluate the Phase 2 trial of bevacizumab in colorectal cancer, which was presented in Chapter 1. This Phase 2 trial enrolled approximately 35 subjects per arm and roughly 23 deaths were observed in each arm of the study. This compares with a total of 385 deaths that were planned for in the following Phase 3 survival trial, which is sufficient to detect a hazard ratio of 0.75 with 80 percent power and type 1 error of 0.025 one sided (Hurwitz et al. 2004). The p-value for the comparison of the 5 mg/kg arm with control in the Phase 2 study was 0.137 two sided or 0.0685 one sided.

The key parameters of a Phase 2 trial design that influence its impact on the efficiency of drug development are f_N and α_2. Now, α_2 is hard to discern from the protocol for a Phase 2 trial since a drug company may choose to move forward with a Phase 3 trial even though the study is not formally positive. But we can calculate the parameter f_N from the number of deaths that were observed in Phase 2 and the number of deaths that were planned for in Phase 3, in this case

$$f_N = \frac{45}{385} = 0.117 \qquad (3.38)$$

When p and α_2 are both less than 0.50, Table 3.3 shows us that this Phase 2/3 program is not dominated by a Phase 3 trial alone. Table 3.4 shows us that if $C/N = 1$, p is less than or equal to 0.20, and α_2 is greater than or equal to 0.05 one sided, then the Phase 2/3 program is admissible; whereas if p is equal to 0.40, then the Phase 2 trial is admissible as long as α_2 is greater than or equal to 0.10 one sided.

To further evaluate the impact of this Phase 2 trial on the efficiency of drug development, Figure 3.5 presents the relative efficiency as a function of f_δ when $f_N = 0.117$, $C/N = 1$, and $p = 0.05$ or $p = 0.20$. $C/N = 1$ is a typical value for a new molecule. Figure 3.5 shows that this Phase 2 trial of bevacizumab will result in a reduction in the efficiency for detecting a treatment with an effect of size $f_\delta = 1$ when α_2 is less than or equal to 0.20 one sided with a greater loss in efficiency with smaller values for α_2. So given the p-value of 0.0685 one sided for the 5 mg/kg arm in this Phase 2 trial, a decision to not continue to Phase 3 as when $\alpha_2 = 0.05$ one sided would result in a substantial decrease in efficiency compared to a Phase 3 trial alone. However, a decision to initiate a Phase 3 trial would be consistent with values for α_2 one sided that are greater than 0.20, values that result in a smaller reduction in efficiency for detecting treatment effects of size $f_\delta = 1$. Indeed, if $\alpha_2 = 0.50$, there will be no reduction in efficiency compared with just doing a Phase 3 trial alone without an accompanying Phase 2 trial. As such, this Phase 2 trial of bevacizumab in colorectal cancer did not help much to improve the efficiency of detecting a treatment effect of the size that the Phase 3 trial was powered to detect.

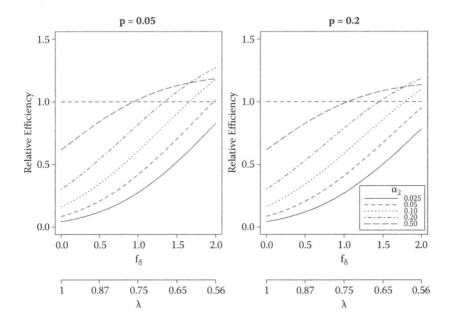

FIGURE 3.5
Relative efficiency for bevacizumab Phase 2 in colorectal cancer. $f_N = 0.117$, $C/N = 1$.

It should be noted that if the goal of the Phase 2/3 program was to discover drugs with a larger treatment effect than the Phase 3 trial was powered to detect, then a larger Phase 2 trial would have greatly improved the efficiency at such treatment effect sizes while reducing the unwanted expense associated with undertaking Phase 3 trials of drugs with small treatment effect sizes. To see this let's take a look at Figure 3.6, which presents the relative efficiency in the circumstances of the bevacizumab Phase 2 trial where we suppose that f_N is equal to 0.30 instead of 0.117 and $\alpha_2 = 0.10$.

By sizing the Phase 2 trial according to $f_N = 0.30$ and testing with $\alpha_2 = 0.10$ one sided we see that the efficiency for detecting drugs with a hazard ratio in the range of 0.50 to 0.65 is much greater than when $f_N = 0.117$ and $\alpha_2 = 0.50$. Although this requires a greater investment upfront in Phase 2 trials, ultimately it will lead to identifying more molecules with the desired treatment effect relative to the investment made in discovering new treatments.

Figure 3.7 presents the numerator of the relative efficiency for the bevacizumab Phase 2 trial along with the numerator of the relative efficiency for the larger Phase 2 trial we have been discussing. Recall that the numerator of the relative efficiency is simply the power of the Phase 2 trial. In Figure 3.7, we see that the power of the Phase 2 trial is less when $f_N = 0.30$ and $\alpha_2 = 0.10$ than when $f_N = 0.117$ and $\alpha_2 = 0.50$. So the probability of initiating Phase 3 with this larger Phase 2 trial is much less than it is with the bevacizumab

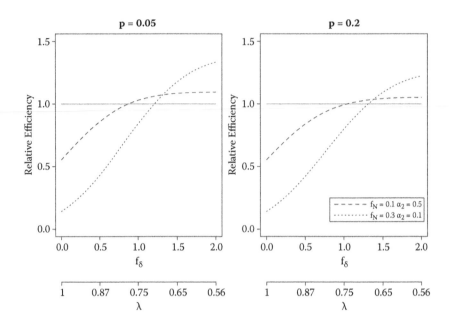

FIGURE 3.6
Relative efficiency for large and small bevacizumab Phase 2 in colorectal cancer. $C/N = 1$.

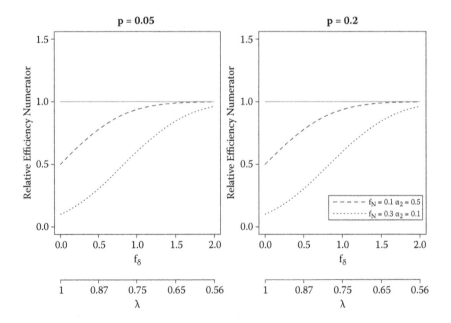

FIGURE 3.7
Numerator of relative efficiency for large and small bevacizumab Phase 2 in colorectal cancer. $C/N = 1$.

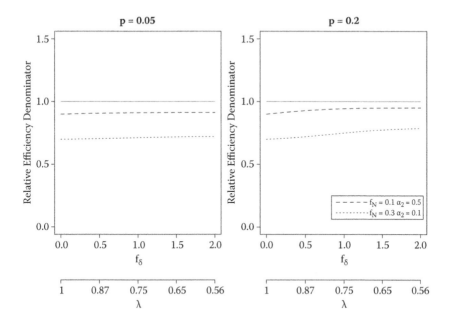

FIGURE 3.8
Denominator of relative efficiency for large and small bevacizumab Phase 2 in colorectal cancer. $C/N = 1$.

Phase 2 trial. However, the denominator of the relative efficiency, which is presented in Figure 3.8 and represents the expected costs of development, is less when $f_N = 0.30$ and $\alpha_2 = 0.10$ than when $f_N = 0.117$ and $\alpha_2 = 0.50$, and this results in a greater efficiency for the large Phase 2 than was observed for the bevacizumab Phase 2 trial.

So larger Phase 2 trials than what was used to evaluate bevacizumab in colorectal cancer will result in fewer drugs with small treatment effects being studied in Phase 3 trials and smaller expected sample sizes. On the whole, more drugs with large treatment effects will be discovered per investment with the large Phase 2 trial investigated in this section.

3.7 Example: Rituximab

This section examines the Phase 2 trial for rituximab in rheumatoid arthritis. The clinical program in rheumatoid arthritis was undertaken after rituximab was approved for use in subjects with relapsed or refractory CD20+, B cell low-grade non-Hodgkin's lymphoma (NHL). Since the initial discovery and development costs for this molecule were covered by the approval in NHL the ratio

C/N may be taken to be zero, reflecting the fact that there are no prior costs to account for in the determination of the efficiency for this clinical program. There were two Phase 2 studies that preceded Phase 3: a Phase 2a study with 40 subjects per arm (Edwards et al. 2004) and a Phase 2b study with approximately 120 subjects per arm that examined two doses of rituximab (Emery et al. 2006). The Phase 3 trial included 300 subjects in the rituximab plus methotrexate arm and 200 in the placebo plus methotrexate arm or roughly 250 subjects per arm (Cohen and Emery 2006). The ACR20 response rate was the primary endpoint in Phase 3, which was powered to detect a difference corresponding to a response rate of 0.45 in the methotrexate plus rituximab arm and a response rate of 0.30 in the methotrexate plus placebo arm.

This example from the rituximab development in rheumatoid arthritis differs from the theory that was developed in this chapter in that there are two Phase 2 trials preceding Phase 3. To account for this we will calculate the efficiency as follows

$$\frac{\Phi\left(z_{\alpha_{2a}} - \left[z_{\alpha_3} - z_\beta\right] \cdot f_\delta \cdot \sqrt{f_{N2a}}\right) \cdot \Phi\left(z_{\alpha_{2b}} - \left[z_{\alpha_3} - z_\beta\right] \cdot f_\delta \cdot \sqrt{f_{N2b}}\right) \cdot \Phi\left(z_{\alpha_3} - \left[z_{\alpha_3} - z_\beta\right] \cdot f_\delta\right)}{C + f_{N2a} + D_1 + D_2}$$

(3.39)

where

$$D_1 = p \cdot \left\{\Phi\left(z_{\alpha_{2a}} - \left[z_{\alpha_3} - z_\beta\right] \cdot f_\delta \cdot \sqrt{f_{N2a}}\right) + (1-p) \cdot \alpha_{2a}\right\} \cdot f_{N2a}$$ (3.40)

and

$$D_2 = p \cdot \left\{\Phi\left(z_{\alpha_{2a}} - \left[z_{\alpha_3} - z_\beta\right] \cdot f_\delta \cdot \sqrt{f_{N2a}}\right) \cdot \Phi\left(z_{\alpha_{2b}} - \left[z_{\alpha_3} - z_\beta\right] \cdot f_\delta \cdot \sqrt{f_{N2b}}\right) + (1-p) \cdot \alpha_{2a} \cdot \alpha_{2b}\right\} \cdot 1$$

(3.41)

For simplicity in presentation we will take $\alpha_{2a} = \alpha_{2b}$.

As before in the bevacizumab example we cannot determine α_{2a} and α_{2b} from the study protocols. We can, however, determine $f_{N2a} = 40 / 250 = 0.16$ for Phase 2a and $f_{N2b} = 120 / 250 = 0.48$ for the Phase 2b. The power in Phase 3 is $\beta = 0.90$.

Figure 3.9 presents the relative efficiency of the Phase 2a and Phase 2b trials for rituximab in rheumatoid arthritis. The figure shows that these Phase 2 trials are able to double the efficiency of a Phase 3 trial alone at the treatment effect size the Phase 3 is powered to detect when α_{2a} and α_{2b} equal 0.20. This differs substantially from the impact of the Phase 2 trial in the bevacizumab example in colorectal cancer and is due primarily to $C/N = 0$ instead of $C/N = 1$ in the bevacizumab Phase 2.

It is interesting to note in Figure 3.9 that the relative efficiency at $\alpha_2 = 0.50$ is less than the relative efficiency at $\alpha_2 = 0.20$ for $f_\delta > 0.75$. In the example of the bevacizumab Phase 2 trial, the relative efficiency at $\alpha_2 = 0.50$ was greater than

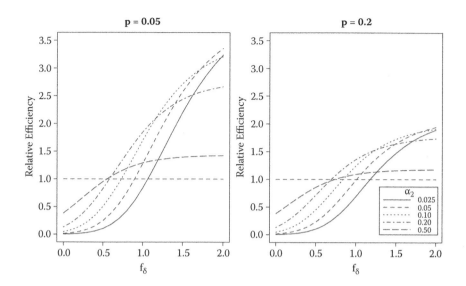

FIGURE 3.9
Relative efficiency for rituximab Phase 2 in rheumatoid arthritis. $f_{N_{2a}} = 0.16$, $f_{N_{2b}} = 0.16$, $C/N = 0$.

the relative efficiency at $\alpha_2 = 0.20$. Further note that the rituximab relative efficiency curves are steeper as the curves move toward and above a relative efficiency of 1. This is at least partly because the additional subjects studied in Phase 2 provide assurance that an active drug with a small treatment effect (e.g., $f_\delta = 0.75$) will not be taken forward to Phase 3.

3.8 Example: TNK

TNK was a thrombolytic developed by Genentech for use in subjects suffering from an acute myocardial infarction. Genentech had already developed a different molecule for this use, namely, TPA, but TNK was designed on the molecular level to be an improved version of TPA.

The primary analysis in Phase 3 was intended to show that the 30-day mortality rate in the TNK group, p_T, was not more than one percent higher than the 30-day mortality rate in the TPA group, p_C (Assent-2 Investigators 1999). If we let δ represent the difference in 30-day mortality between TNK and TPA that has to be ruled out, that is, one percent, and we let θ represent the true difference in mortality rates between the two arms then we can write the power for this analysis as

$$P\left(\frac{\hat{p}_T - \hat{p}_C - \delta}{\sqrt{\hat{p}_T \cdot \hat{q}_T / N + \hat{p}_C \cdot \hat{q}_C / N}} < z_\alpha\right) = \beta \qquad (3.42)$$

or

$$P\left(Z < z_\alpha + \frac{\delta - \theta}{\sqrt{\hat{p}_T \cdot \hat{q}_T / N + \hat{p}_C \cdot \hat{q}_C / N}}\right) = \beta \qquad (3.43)$$

Now since

$$z_\alpha + \frac{\delta - \theta}{\sqrt{\hat{p}_T \cdot \hat{q}_T / N + \hat{p}_C \cdot \hat{q}_C / N}} = z_\beta \qquad (3.44)$$

$$z_\alpha - z_\beta = (-1) \cdot \frac{(\delta - \theta)}{\sqrt{\hat{p}_T \cdot \hat{q}_T / N + \hat{p}_C \cdot \hat{q}_C / N}} \qquad (3.45)$$

we can rewrite the power as

$$P\left(Z < z_\alpha - \left[z_\alpha - z_\beta\right] \cdot f_{\theta-\delta} \cdot \sqrt{f_N}\right) \qquad (3.46)$$

Thus, we may write the relative efficiency again as

$$\frac{\Phi\left(z_{\alpha_2} - \left[z_{\alpha_3} - z_\beta\right] \cdot f_{\theta-\delta} \cdot \sqrt{f_N}\right)}{\left\{f_N + p \cdot \Phi\left(z_{\alpha_2} - \left[z_{\alpha_3} - z_\beta\right] \cdot f_{\theta-\delta} \cdot \sqrt{f_N}\right) + (1-p) \cdot \alpha_2 + \frac{C}{N}\right\} \cdot \frac{N}{C+N}} \qquad (3.47)$$

Since TPA had already been shown to reduce 30-day mortality and TNK was designed to be more effective at hitting the same target than TPA and since other molecules that break up clots also had demonstrated a benefit on 30-day mortality in this patient population, there was relatively high confidence that TNK would meet or exceed the regulatory requirements for showing noninferiority to TPA on the endpoint of 30-day mortality.

There was, however, more uncertainty and concern over whether the intracranial hemorrhage (ICH) rate for TNK would be too high since it was designed to be more effective at breaking up clots than TPA. In this regard, it is also interesting to note that the size of the treatment effect for ICH was greater than the size of the treatment effect for 30-day mortality. Specifically, the treatment effect for 30-day mortality in a two-arm comparative trial is

$$\frac{0.01}{\sqrt{2 \cdot 0.06 \cdot 0.94}} = 0.0298 \qquad (3.48)$$

whereas the treatment effect for ICH in a single-arm historically controlled study is

$$\frac{0.015 - 0.007}{\sqrt{0.015 \cdot 0.995}} = 0.655 \tag{3.49}$$

In the Phase 2 trial for TNK to study ICH, the 30-day mortality rate was expected to be around 6 percent (Van de Werf and Cannon 1999). The ICH rate observed in the Gusto trial was 0.7 percent (Gusto Investigators 1993) and an increase in the ICH rate to a level of 1.5 percent or more in this Phase 2 trial was judged to be not acceptable.

Both the increased uncertainty and treatment effect size for the ICH rate compared with the 30-day mortality rate imply Phase 2 would provide greater efficiency for finding a drug that meets the objective for ICH than the objective for 30-day mortality. Figure 3.10 shows that the efficiency of development for 30-day mortality whether p is 0.20, 0.50, or 0.75 is very close to one and thus a randomized Phase 2 trial looking at 30-day mortality does not help much to ensure the Phase 3 trial achieves its objectives on that endpoint.

However, in terms of ensuring that the Phase 3 study meets its objectives concerning the ICH rate, there is a notable improvement in efficiency that results from this Phase 2 trial. This provides a nice justification for the ASSENT-1 trial, which was the Phase 2 trial of TNK to evaluate its effect on ICH rates. Here we are ignoring potential biases that may result from the fact that the Phase 2 trial used historical controls. We will address historical controlled trials in Chapter 5.

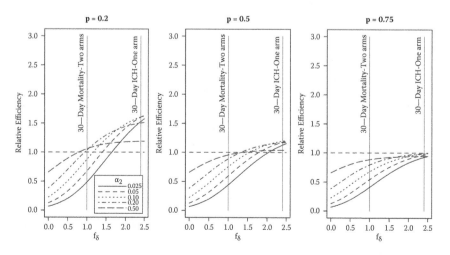

FIGURE 3.10
Relative efficiency for TNK Phase 2 in acute myocardial infarction. $f_N = 0.20$, $C/N = 0.25$.

3.9 Summary

This chapter showed that when looking only at the efficiency of a Phase 2 and Phase 3 clinical trial program, Phase 2 trials can substantially improve the efficiency with which active drugs are identified and proven to be so in Phase 3. However, when accounting for the costs of drug discovery, that is, when trying to optimize the drug development process as a whole, Phase 2 screening trials provide little benefit over simply doing a Phase 3 trial without a preceding Phase 2 screening trial, even if the true magnitude of the treatment effect is 50 percent greater than what one would assume in planning a Phase 3 clinical trial. So although it may be appropriate to conduct Phase 2 screening trials when there are a lot of candidates that have completed Phase 1 and not enough money to study them all in Phase 3, it is not a good strategy for a drug company to push a large number of drugs into clinical development to be screened with underpowered Phase 2 clinical studies unless the present value of the associated discovery costs are a small fraction of the Phase 2/3 development costs.

References

Assent-2 Investigators. 1999. Single-bolus tenecteplase compared with front-loaded alteplase in acute myocardial infarction: The ASSENT-2 double-blind randomised trial. *Lancet* 354:716–722.

Cannon, C.P., Gibson, C. M., et al. 1998. TNK-tissue plasminogen activator compared with front-loaded alteplase in acute myocardial infarction: Results of the TIMI 10B trial. *Circulation* 98:2805–2814.

Cohen, S.B., Emery. P. 2006. Rituximab for Rheumatoid Arthritis Refractory to anti-tumor necrosis factor therapy—Results of a multicenter, randomized, double-blind, placebo-controlled, phase III trial evaluating primary efficacy and safety at twenty-four weeks. *Arthritis Rheum* 54(9):2793–2806.

DiMasi, J.A., Hansen, R.W., Grabowski, H.G 2003. The price of innovation: New estimates of drug development costs. *J Health Econ* 22:151–185.

Edwards, J.C.W., Szczepanski, L., et al. 2004. Efficacy of B-cell-targeted therapy with rituximab in rheumatoid arthritis. *N Engl J Med* 350:2572–2581.

Emery, P., Fleischmann R., et al. 2006. The efficacy and safety of rituximab in patients with active rheumatoid arthritis despite methotrexate treatment—Results of a Phase IIb randomized, double-blind, placebo-controlled, dose-ranging trial. *Arthritis Rheum* 54(5):1390–1400.

Gusto Investigators. 1993. An international randomized trial comparing four thrombolytic strategies for acute myocardial infarction. *N Engl J Med* 329:673–682.

Holmgren, E.B. 2008. Are Phase 2 screening trials in oncology obsolete? *Stat Med* 27(4):556–567.

Hurwitz, H., Fehrenbacher, L., et al. 2004. Bevacizumab plus irinotecan, fluorouracil, and leucovorin for metastatic colorectal cancer. *N Engl J Med* 350:2335–2342.

Van de Werf, F., Cannon, C.P. 1999. Safety assessment of single-bolus administration of TNK tissue-plasminogen activator in acute myocardial infarction: The ASSENT-1 trial. *Am Heart J* 137:786–791.

Wald, A. 1947. An essentially complete class of admissible decision functions. *Ann Math Statist* 18(4):549–555.

4

Maximize the Minimum Efficiency

In the previous chapter, we constructed an admissible class of Phase 2 trial designs and decision rules to help guide the design of Phase 2 trials and the associated decision making. In this section we consider another approach to designing the Phase 2/3 clinical development program for a new drug which is to maximize the minimum efficiency. That is, taking the magnitude of the treatment effect as uncertain, one could proceed to design the Phase 2 trial in such a way as to minimize the impact on efficiency if the magnitude of the treatment effect turns out to be the worst case for efficiency.

In this chapter we show that a clinical development program consisting only of a Phase 3 trial with no accompanying Phase 2 trial maximizes the minimum relative efficiency and then that it maximizes the minimum efficiency. To see this, first note that the relative efficiency decreases as f_δ decreases to zero. This follows since the derivative of the relative efficiency with respect to f_δ is greater than zero as shown in Equations (4.1) through (4.3).

$$\frac{\partial}{\partial f_\delta} \frac{\Phi(a)}{\left[f_N + p \cdot \Phi(a) + (1-p)\alpha_2 + C/N \right] \cdot N/(C+N)}$$

$$= \frac{C+N}{N} \left(\left[f_N + p \cdot \Phi(a) + (1-p) \cdot \alpha_2 + C/N \right] \cdot \frac{\partial \Phi(a)}{\partial f_\delta} - \Phi(a) \cdot p \cdot \frac{\partial \Phi(a)}{\partial f_\delta} \right) \frac{1}{K^2}$$

$$\tag{4.1}$$

$$= \frac{C+N}{N} \left[f_N + (1-p) \cdot \alpha_2 + C/N \right] \cdot \frac{\partial \Phi(a)}{\partial f_\delta} \frac{1}{K^2} \tag{4.2}$$

$$= \frac{C+N}{N} \left[f_N + (1-p) \cdot \alpha_2 + C/N \right] \cdot \varphi(a)(-1)(z_{\alpha_3} - z_\beta)\sqrt{f_N} \frac{1}{K^2} > 0 \tag{4.3}$$

where $a = z_{\alpha_2} - \left[z_{\alpha_3} - z_\beta \right] \cdot f_\delta \cdot \sqrt{f_N}$ and

$$K = \left[f_N + p \cdot \Phi(a) + (1-p)\alpha_2 + C/N \right] \tag{4.4}$$

The last inequality holds since $z_{\alpha_3} < z_\beta$.

Next note that the limit of the relative efficiency as f_δ decreases to zero is less than one. To see this first observe that

$$\lim_{f\delta\to 0} \frac{\Phi(a)}{\left[f_N + p\cdot\Phi(a) + (1-p)\alpha_2 + C/N\right]\cdot N/(C+N)}$$

$$= \frac{\alpha_2}{\left(f_N + \alpha_2 + C/N\right)\cdot N/(C+N)} \tag{4.5}$$

Now

$$\frac{\alpha_2}{\left(f_N + \alpha_2 + C/N\right)\cdot N/(C+N)} < 1 \tag{4.6}$$

if and only if

$$\frac{C+N}{N}\cdot\alpha_2 < f_N + \alpha_2 + \frac{C}{N} \tag{4.7}$$

if and only if

$$\frac{C}{N}\cdot\alpha_2 < f_N + \frac{C}{N} \tag{4.8}$$

which is true since $0 < \alpha_2 < 1$ and $f_N > 0$.

Finally note that by definition, the relative efficiency of a Phase 3 trial alone is one. This can also be seen by taking the limit of the relative efficiency as $\alpha_2 \to 1$ and $f_N \to 0$.

$$\lim_{\substack{\alpha_2\to 1 \\ f_N\to 0}} \frac{\Phi(a)}{\left[f_N + p\cdot\Phi(a) + (1-p)\alpha_2 + C/N\right]\cdot N/(C+N)}$$

$$= \frac{1}{\left(0 + p + (1-p) + C/N\right)\cdot\dfrac{N}{C+N}} = 1 \tag{4.9}$$

This shows that a Phase 3 trial alone maximizes the minimum relative efficiency for $f_\delta > 0$ among all Phase 2 trials and decision rules represented by $H = \{(\alpha_2, f_N): 0 < \alpha_2 < 1 \text{ and } f_N > 0\}$.

The result that a Phase 3 trial alone maximizes the minimum efficiency follows by noting that the efficiency of a Phase 3 trial decreases as f_δ decreases to zero.

$$\frac{\partial}{\partial f_\delta}\frac{\Phi(a)}{N+C} = \frac{\phi(a)}{N+C}\cdot(-1)\cdot(z_{\alpha_2} - z_\beta)\cdot\sqrt{f_N} > 0 \tag{4.10}$$

So, since the relative efficiency of any Phase 2 trial in H and the efficiency of a Phase 3 trial alone decrease as $f_\delta \downarrow 0$, the efficiency of a Phase 2/3 development program decreases as $f_\delta \downarrow 0$ for all $\langle \alpha_2, f_N \rangle \in H$ and hence the minimum is achieved as $f_\delta \downarrow 0$. This is also where the strategy that includes just a Phase 3 trial maximizes the minimum relative efficiency among all $\langle \alpha_2, f_N \rangle \in H$. Thus, a Phase 2/3 clinical development strategy that includes only a Phase 3 trial will maximize the minimum efficiency.

This result shows that a Phase 3 trial alone is the strategy that will maximize the minimum relative efficiency. In particular, when the treatment effect size, f_δ, is small the Phase 3 trial alone will be close to the strategy that will maximize the efficiency.

5

Single-Arm Phase 2 Trial

The preceding development of the efficiency of a Phase 2/3 clinical program did not address the use of a single-arm Phase 2 trial, that is, a Phase 2 trial without a control arm. The concern with using a single arm Phase 2 trial in a quantitative approach to identifying active drugs is that it is susceptible to selection bias, which can make the study results uninterpretable. In particular, selection bias can make a drug that is no different than a placebo appear to have promising activity. Here we present an approach to using Phase 2 single-arm trials that account for potential selection bias.

Suppose that it is known that subjects treated with the standard of care have a response that is normally distributed with mean μ_C and variance σ^2. Further, let p represent the proportion of eligible patients at the site who were enrolled in a study. If the patients who were most likely to achieve the best responses were selected for entry into the trial, then the expected response would be

$$\frac{\int\limits_{-\infty}^{a} x \frac{1}{\sigma} \phi\left(\frac{x-\mu_C}{\sigma}\right) \cdot dx}{\int\limits_{-\infty}^{a} \frac{1}{\sigma} \phi\left(\frac{x-\mu_C}{\sigma}\right) \cdot dx} = \frac{\int\limits_{-\infty}^{(a-\mu_C)/\sigma} \sigma y \phi(y) \cdot dy}{\int\limits_{-\infty}^{(a-\mu_C)/\sigma} \phi(y) \cdot dy} + \mu_C \tag{5.1}$$

$$= \frac{\sigma}{\Phi\left(\frac{a-\mu_C}{\sigma}\right)} \int\limits_{-\infty}^{(a-\mu_C)/\sigma} y \phi(y) \cdot dy + \mu_C \tag{5.2}$$

Here

$$p = \int\limits_{-\infty}^{a} \frac{1}{\sigma} \phi\left(\frac{x-\mu_C}{\sigma}\right) \cdot dx \tag{5.3}$$

If we let responses under the alternative be normally distributed with mean μ_T and variance σ^2, then the power of the study to detect a treatment effect over and above any potential selection bias will be

$$P\left(\dfrac{\bar{X}-\left[\mu_C+\dfrac{\sigma}{\Phi\big([a-\mu_C]/\sigma\big)}\displaystyle\int_{-\infty}^{(a-\mu_C)/\sigma} y\,\phi(y)\cdot dy\right]}{\sqrt{\sigma^2/n}}<z_\alpha\right)$$

$$=P\left(\dfrac{\bar{X}-\mu_T-\left[\mu_C+\dfrac{\sigma}{\Phi\big([a-\mu_C]/\sigma\big)}\displaystyle\int_{-\infty}^{(a-\mu_C)/\sigma} y\,\phi(y)\cdot dy\right]}{\sqrt{\sigma^2/n}}<z_\alpha-\dfrac{\mu_T}{\sqrt{\sigma^2/n}}\right) \qquad (5.4)$$

$$=P\left(\dfrac{\bar{X}-\mu_T}{\sqrt{\sigma^2/n}}<z_\alpha-\dfrac{\mu_T-\mu_C-\dfrac{\sigma}{\Phi\big([a-\mu_C]/\sigma\big)}\displaystyle\int_{-\infty}^{(a-\mu_C)/\sigma} y\,\phi(y)\cdot dy}{\sqrt{\sigma^2/n}}\right) \qquad (5.5)$$

$$=\Phi\left(z_\alpha-\dfrac{\mu_T-\mu_C-\dfrac{\sigma}{\Phi\big([a-\mu_C]/\sigma\big)}\displaystyle\int_{-\infty}^{(a-\mu_C)/\sigma} y\,\phi(y)\cdot dy}{\sqrt{\sigma^2/n}}\right) \qquad (5.6)$$

The ratio of the treatment effect size in a single-arm Phase 2 over and above the potential selection bias to the treatment effect size for the Phase 3 trial is

$$\dfrac{\dfrac{\mu_T-\mu_C-\dfrac{\sigma}{\Phi\big([a-\mu_C]/\sigma\big)}\displaystyle\int_{-\infty}^{(a-\mu_C)/\sigma} y\,\phi(y)\cdot dy}{\sqrt{\sigma^2}}}{\dfrac{(\mu_T-\mu_C)}{\sqrt{2\sigma^2}}} \qquad (5.7)$$

$$=\sqrt{2}\left[1-\dfrac{\sigma}{\mu_T-\mu_C}\dfrac{1}{\Phi\big([a-\mu_C]/\sigma\big)}\displaystyle\int_{-\infty}^{(a-\mu_C)/\sigma} y\,\phi(y)\cdot dy\right]=f_\delta$$

As the proportion of eligible subjects enrolled in the trial converges to zero, that is, as $p \to 0$ then $(a - \mu_C)/\sigma \to -\infty$ and so $f_\delta \to -\infty$. On the other hand, as $p \to 1$, $(a - \mu_C)/\sigma \to +\infty$ and f_δ converges to

$$\lim_{p \to 1} \sqrt{2}\left[1 - \frac{\sigma}{\mu_T - \mu_C} \cdot \frac{1}{p} \int_{-\infty}^{(a-\mu_C)/\sigma} y\phi(y) \cdot dy\right]$$

$$= \sqrt{2}\left[1 - \frac{\sigma}{\mu_T - \mu_C} \cdot \int_{-\infty}^{\infty} y\phi(y) \cdot dy\right] \tag{5.8}$$

$$= \sqrt{2}[1 - 0] = \sqrt{2} \tag{5.9}$$

Figure 5.1 provides a graph of $\dfrac{1}{p} \displaystyle\int_{-\infty}^{(a-\mu_C)/\sigma} y\phi(y)$. Figure 5.1 shows that if the probability of selection is less than $0.\overline{5}$, then the value of $\dfrac{1}{p} \displaystyle\int_{-\infty}^{(a-\mu_C)/\sigma} y\phi(y)$ will be less than –1. So, if $\sigma/(\mu_T - \mu_C)$ is also less than –1, then f_δ will be negative, that is, the single-arm Phase 2 study will not detect a treatment effect regardless of the sample size. The larger p is the more negative $\sigma/(\mu_T - \mu_C)$ may be and still result in a trial that can detect a treatment effect over and above

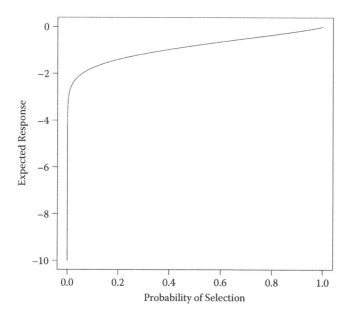

FIGURE 5.1
Graph of the expected response under patient selection. $\mu_C = 0$, $\sigma = 1$.

any potential selection bias. In other words, the larger p is the smaller the magnitude of the treatment effect that can be detected after accounting for potential selection bias. f_δ determined in this way can be used in the formulas and tables for relative efficiency in the previous chapter.

So, a Phase 2 single-arm trial that enrolls all eligible subjects will have more power than a randomized Phase 2 trial with the same number of subjects. However, enrollment of a fraction of the eligible patients into the trial can substantially degrade the usefulness of such a trial in drug development. The key to a single-arm trial improving efficiency over a randomized trial is that there be little or no selection bias. A simple way to ensure this is to require that everyone who is eligible for a trial at a site is enrolled. The practice of a site having several studies open and guiding patients to the study perceived to be the best for the patient leaves a single-arm trial susceptible to selection bias and is not a practice consistent with promoting the discovery of active drugs for the benefit of future patients.

6

Phase 2 Trials Based on Surrogate Endpoints

Until now, we have evaluated the impact of a Phase 2 trial on the efficiency of the drug development process when the primary endpoint of the Phase 2 study is also the primary endpoint in Phase 3. However, in many clinical trial settings, surrogates are used in Phase 2 in place of the primary endpoint for Phase 3. For example, tumor response and progression free survival are often used as surrogates for survival in oncology trials. This section evaluates the impact on the efficiency of drug development of a Phase 2 screening trial whose primary endpoint is a surrogate variable for the Phase 3 primary endpoint.

Prentice (1989) developed a criteria for a variable S to be a surrogate of another variable T, which is summarized in the following four statements

$$f(S|Z) \neq f(S) \tag{6.1}$$

$$f(T|Z) \neq f(T) \tag{6.2}$$

$$f(T|S) \neq f(T) \tag{6.3}$$

$$f(T|S,Z) = f(T|S) \tag{6.4}$$

Here, Z is an indicator for treatment. These statements imply that the effect of treatment, represented by Z, on the variable T is completely accounted for by the surrogate S.

A surrogate variable as defined by Prentice (1989) is very hard to find. There are very few if any examples of variables that are true surrogates as so defined. That does not mean that variables that are not surrogates but are associated with a Phase 3 primary endpoint cannot still help improve the efficiency of drug development. We will use the term surrogate in this section not in the sense of Prentice but in the sense that a variable is associated with another variable that is used as a Phase 3 primary endpoint for regulatory approval. In this chapter we evaluate the impact of a "surrogate" variable on the efficiency of drug development and set out an empirical approach to developing and using surrogate variables in drug development.

6.1 Impact of a Surrogate on the Efficiency of Drug Development

To start this investigation of the impact of a surrogate on the efficiency of drug development, we need to specify a relationship between the surrogate and its associated Phase 3 endpoint. Suppose that relationship is given simply by

$$\mu = a + b \cdot \theta \tag{6.5}$$

where μ represents the Phase 3 endpoint and θ represents the value of the surrogate. Let $\theta_{T,0}$ and $\theta_{T,1}$ denote, respectively, the expected baseline and postbaseline values for the surrogate in the experimental treatment group. Likewise, let $\theta_{C,0}$ and $\theta_{C,1}$ denote the same quantities for the control group. Define $\Delta\theta_T = \theta_{T,1} - \theta_{T,0}$ and $\Delta\theta_C = \theta_{C,1} - \theta_{C,0}$. Then the relationship between the Z-statistic for the drug's effect on the surrogate and the Z-statistic for the drug's effect on the associated Phase 3 endpoint is

$$\frac{\Delta\theta_T - \Delta\theta_C}{\sqrt{2\sigma_{\Delta\theta}^2/n_{\Delta\theta}}} = \frac{\Delta\mu_T - \Delta\mu_C - \tau}{b \cdot \sqrt{2\sigma_{\Delta\theta}^2/n_{\Delta\theta}}} \tag{6.6}$$

$$= \frac{\Delta\mu_T - \Delta\mu_C}{b \cdot \sqrt{2\sigma_{\Delta\mu}^2/n_{\Delta\mu}}} \frac{\sqrt{2\sigma_{\Delta\mu}^2/n_{\Delta\mu}}}{\sqrt{2\sigma_{\Delta\theta}^2/n_{\Delta\theta}}} - \frac{\tau}{b \cdot \sqrt{2\sigma_{\Delta\theta}^2/n_{\Delta\theta}}}$$

$$= \frac{\Delta\mu_T - \Delta\mu_C}{\sqrt{2\sigma_{\Delta\mu}^2/n_{\Delta\mu}}} \cdot \frac{\sigma_{\Delta\mu}}{b \cdot \sigma_{\Delta\theta}} \cdot \sqrt{\frac{n_{\Delta\theta}}{n_{\Delta\mu}}} - x \tag{6.7}$$

where

$$x \sim N\left(0, \frac{\sigma_\tau^2}{2 \cdot b^2 \sigma_\theta^2/n_\theta}\right) \tag{6.8}$$

Here, τ represents a random effect that allows the relationship between the surrogate variable and its associated Phase 3 endpoint to not be exactly linear.

With this notation, the power of a Phase 2 trial with a surrogate variable as the primary endpoint, which we will denote by Π, can be expressed as follows

$$\Pi = P\left(\frac{\Delta\theta_T - \Delta\theta_C}{\sqrt{2 \cdot \sigma_\theta^2/n_{\Delta\theta}}} < z_{\alpha 2}\right) \tag{6.9}$$

$$
= \int\limits_{-\infty}^{\infty} \left\{ \begin{array}{l} \Phi\left(z_{\alpha_2} - \dfrac{\Delta\mu_T - \Delta\mu_C}{\sqrt{2 \cdot \sigma_\mu^2 / n_{\Delta\mu}}} \cdot \dfrac{\sigma_{\Delta\mu}}{b \cdot \sigma_{\Delta\theta}} \cdot \sqrt{\dfrac{n_{\Delta\theta}}{n_{\Delta\mu}}} - x \right) \\[4mm] \times \phi\left(x \cdot b \cdot \left[\dfrac{2 \cdot \sigma_{\Delta\theta}^2 / n_{\Delta\theta}}{\sigma_\tau^2} \right]^{1/2} \right) \cdot b \left[\dfrac{2 \cdot \sigma_{\Delta\theta}^2 / n_{\Delta\theta}}{\sigma_\tau^2} \right]^{1/2} \end{array} \right\} \cdot dx \qquad (6.10)
$$

Here, $\sigma_{\Delta\theta}^2$ represents the variance of the surrogate $\Delta\theta$, $\sigma_{\Delta\mu}^2$ represents the variance of the Phase 3 summary statistic $\Delta\mu$, $n_{\Delta\theta}$ represents the number of subjects/events in each of the experimental and control groups in Phase 2 that is relevant for determining the power of the surrogate, $n_{\Delta\mu}$ represents the number of subjects/events in each of the experimental and control groups in Phase 2 that is relevant for determining the power of the Phase 3 endpoint, and z_{α_2} represents the level of testing in Phase 2.

Note that in the situation where the Phase 3 endpoint is a time to event variable and the treatment and control groups are determined by randomization, we may write

$$
\Delta\mu_T - \Delta\mu_C = \mu_{T,1} - \mu_{C,1} = \log(\lambda_T) - \log(\lambda_C) \qquad (6.11)
$$

That is, we may take $\Delta\mu$ to be the log hazard and σ_μ^2 to be the variance of the log hazard.

If we use the data collected on the surrogate in Phase 2 to make the decision whether to go forward with a Phase 3 trial then the efficiency of drug development becomes

$$
\frac{p \cdot \Pi \cdot \Phi\left(z_{\alpha_3} - \left[z_{\alpha_3} - z_\beta \right] \cdot f_\delta \right)}{C + n + N \cdot \left[p \cdot \Pi + (1 - p) \cdot \alpha_2 \right]} \qquad (6.12)
$$

where Π is defined as in Equation (6.10). Factoring out the efficiency of a Phase 3 trial alone, the remaining quantity is the relative efficiency of drug development

$$
\frac{\Pi}{\left\{ p \cdot \Pi + (1 - p) \cdot \alpha_2 + \dfrac{C + n}{N} \right\} \cdot \dfrac{N}{C + N}} \qquad (6.13)
$$

If the relative efficiency is greater than one, we can say that a development program that incorporates the surrogate in a Phase 2 screening trial is more efficient than a development program without a Phase 2 screening trial. On the other hand, if the relative efficiency is less than one, then a Phase 3 study without a preceding Phase 2 trial is more efficient.

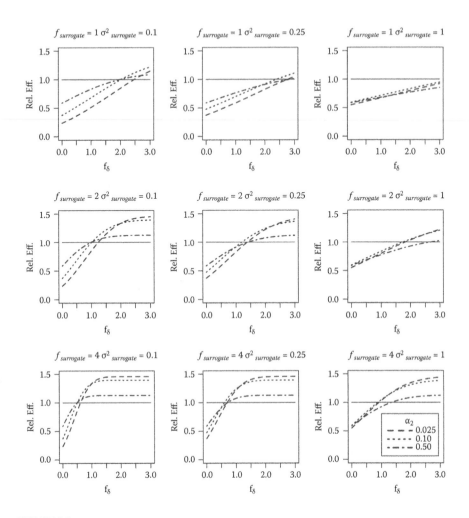

FIGURE 6.1
Efficiency of a Phase 2 screening trial of a surrogate endpoint for the Phase 3 primary endpoint.

Figure 6.1 illustrates how the relative efficiency changes as $f_{Surrogate} = \dfrac{\sigma_\mu}{b \cdot \sigma_\theta}$ and $\sigma^2_{Surrogate} = \dfrac{\sigma^2_\tau}{b^2 \cdot \sigma^2_\theta}$ change. Specifically, the panels present the relative efficiency for $f_{Surrogate}$ assuming values of 1, 2, and 4, and $\sigma^2_{Surrogate}$ assuming values of 0.1, 0.25, and 1.0. In Figure 6.1, the probability that the drug is active, p, is assumed to be 0.20, b as used in Equation (6.9) is taken to be 1, and there are 50 subjects in each arm of the Phase 2 study with 60 events total (30 per arm). The type 1 error for testing for the difference between two groups in Phase 2 is evaluated at three levels: 0.50, 0.10, and 0.025 one sided. f_N is 0.15 and C is set equal to N since capitalized pre-Phase 2 development costs are roughly equal to capitalized Phase 3 development costs.

In every panel of Figure 6.1, as $f_{Surrogate}$ increases from one, the relative efficiency increases as well. Further, increases in $\sigma_{Surrogate}$ result in a flattening of the relative efficiency curve. Increasing α_2 decreases the maximum improvement in efficiency that is possible. The figures demonstrate that in this particular example there is the potential for a biomarker to substantially improve the efficiency of drug development.

6.2 Estimation of the Potential Impact of a Specific Surrogate on Efficiency

Now that we have shown there is a potential to substantially improve the efficiency of drug development by using a surrogate in Phase 2, we turn to the question of how to identify such a surrogate. So, suppose that there are at hand N randomized Phase 2 studies that evaluate the effect of N different experimental treatments on a particular surrogate and survival. Note that it is not uncommon for subjects to be followed for survival in such a Phase 2 trial, even though survival may not be a primary endpoint.

The data that are available to estimate the relative efficiency are the difference between groups in the mean change in the surrogate from baseline, $\Delta\hat{\theta}_{T,i} - \Delta\hat{\theta}_{C,i}, i = 1, \ldots, N$, the log hazard ratio as estimated from the Cox model, $\log(\hat{\lambda}_{T,i}/\hat{\lambda}_{C,i}), i = 1, \ldots, N$ and $\Delta\hat{\theta}_{T,i} - \Delta\hat{\theta}_{C,i}$. Note that $\Delta\hat{\theta}_{T,i} - \Delta\hat{\theta}_{C,i}$ and $\log(\hat{\lambda}_{T,i}/\hat{\lambda}_{C,i})$ are jointly distributed as

$$\begin{vmatrix} \Delta\hat{\theta}_{T,i} - \Delta\hat{\theta}_{C,i} \\ \log(\hat{\lambda}_{T,i}/\hat{\lambda}_{C,i}) \end{vmatrix} \sim N\left(\begin{bmatrix} \Delta\theta_{T,i} - \Delta\theta_{C,i} \\ b \cdot (\Delta\theta_{T,i} - \Delta\theta_{C,i}) \end{bmatrix}, \begin{bmatrix} 2 \cdot \sigma_\theta^2/n_i & 0 \\ 0 & 1/d_{T,i} + 1/d_{C,i} + \sigma_\tau^2 \end{bmatrix} \right) \quad (6.14)$$

and the variance of $\Delta\hat{\theta}_{T,i} - \Delta\hat{\theta}_{C,i}$ is independently distributed as

$$\text{var}\left(\Delta\hat{\theta}_{T,i} - \Delta\hat{\theta}_{C,i} \right) \sim \chi_{2n_i-2}^2 \cdot \frac{\sigma_\theta^2}{2n_i - 2} \quad (6.15)$$

The statistics from study i are independent of the statistics from study j, where $i \neq j$. Here, $d_{T,i}$ and $d_{C,i}$ represent the number of deaths observed in the experimental treatment and control arms of study i, $i = 1\ldots N$.

The diagonal of the variance covariance matrix is determined as follows. The first diagonal element is the variance of the sample estimate of $\Delta\theta_{T,i} - \Delta\theta_{C,i}$

and so is simply $2 \cdot \sigma_\theta^2/n_i$. The second diagonal element is $\mathrm{var}\left(\log(\hat{\lambda}_{T,i}/\hat{\lambda}_{C,i})\right)$. Now since $\Delta\theta_{T,i} - \Delta\theta_{C,i}$ is linearly related to the true hazard ratio with error contributed by a random effect with variance σ_τ^2, the second diagonal element is σ_τ^2, plus the variance in estimating the log of the hazard ratio from the Cox model, $1/d_{T,i} + 1/d_{C,i}$. For simplicity and ease of presentation, we take the correlation between the errors in estimating $\Delta\theta_{T,i} - \Delta\theta_{C,i}$ and the errors in estimating $\log(\lambda_{T,i}/(\lambda_{C,i})$ to be zero, which makes the off diagonals of the variance covariance matrix zero. While this assumption is reasonable, it can be relaxed as is appropriate.

Now note that this model is parameterized by b, $\Delta\theta_{T,i} - \Delta\theta_{C,i}$, σ_θ^2, and σ_τ^2. However, to determine the relative efficiency of a surrogate we just need estimates for b and σ_τ^2. The parameters $\Delta\theta_{T,i} - \Delta\theta_{C,i}$ and σ_θ^2 simply describe the properties of the surrogate in a particular study and so are nuisance parameters when it comes to estimating the relationship between a surrogate and survival, which is what we need to estimate the efficiency of a surrogate.

To estimate the parameters b, σ_τ^2, σ_θ^2, and $\Delta\theta_{T,i} - \Delta\theta_{C,i}$ we use maximum likelihood implemented with a two-stage iterative process. The essence of this two-stage process is described in Equations (6.16) and (6.17), which are solutions for $\Delta\theta_{T,i} - \Delta\theta_{C,i}$ and σ_θ^2 from their respective derivatives of the log likelihood function.

$$\Delta\theta_{T,i} - \Delta\theta_{C,i} = \frac{\dfrac{b^2}{1/d_{T,i} + 1/d_{C,i} + \sigma_\tau^2} \cdot \dfrac{\log(\hat{\lambda}_{T,i}/\hat{\lambda}_{C,i})}{b} + \dfrac{1}{2\sigma_\theta^2/n_i} \cdot \left(\Delta\hat{\theta}_{T,i} - \Delta\hat{\theta}_{C,i}\right)}{\dfrac{b^2}{1/d_{T,i} + 1/d_{C,i} + \sigma_\tau^2} + \dfrac{1}{2\sigma_\theta^2/n_i}} \tag{6.16}$$

$$\sigma_\theta^2 = \sum_{i=1}^{N} \frac{\left[\Delta\hat{\theta}_{T,i} - \Delta\hat{\theta}_{C,i} - \left(\Delta\theta_{T,i} - \Delta\theta_{C,i}\right)\right]^2}{2 \cdot N} \tag{6.17}$$

So, if we are given initial values for the parameters σ_θ^2 and $\Delta\theta_{T,i} - \Delta\theta_{C,i}$ we can create estimates for the parameters b and σ_τ^2 by maximizing the log likelihood function with respect to b and σ_τ^2. Using these estimates for b and σ_τ^2 we can estimate σ_θ^2 and $\Delta\theta_{T,i} - \Delta\theta_{C,i}$ using Equations (6.16) and (6.17). This process can continue until the estimates converge.

Using the techniques of maximum likelihood we can create a variance–covariance matrix for all the parameter estimates. The key parameters we need to estimate the efficiency are b and σ_τ^2. These parameters relate the information about the surrogate in a specific study to the estimates effect on survival. To calculate the uncertainty in the relative efficiency we use the following equation along with the estimates and the associated variance covariance matrix of the parameters b and σ_τ^2

$$\text{var(Rel Eff)} = \left(\frac{\partial \text{ Rel Eff.}}{\partial b} \right)^2 \cdot \text{var}(b) + \left(\frac{\partial \text{ Rel. Eff.}}{\partial \sigma_\tau} \right)^2 \cdot \text{var}(\sigma_\tau)$$
$$+ \frac{\partial \text{ Rel Eff.}}{\partial b} \cdot \frac{\partial \text{ Rel. Eff.}}{\partial \sigma_\tau} \cdot \text{cov}(b, \sigma_\tau) \tag{6.18}$$

Holmgren (2008) gives more details on the maximum likelihood estimates and the variance–covariance matrix for the parameters.

Figure 6.3 presents the relative efficiency of a Phase 2 screening trial where progression free survival (PFS) is used as a surrogate for survival. The data to support Figure 6.3, which are presented in Figure 6.2, are from the paper by Buyse et al. (2007). Thirteen studies in colorectal cancer evaluating the treatment benefit of FU + LV, FU, irinotecan, and oxaliplatin were included. Note that the evaluation of this data tells us how PFS predicts overall survival (OS) across different study populations instead of across different molecules. The 90 percent confidence interval around the relative efficiency curve excludes the efficiency curve of a Phase 2 screening

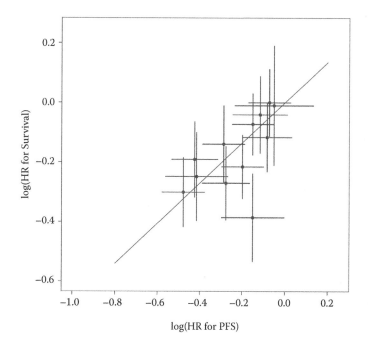

FIGURE 6.2
Hazard ratio for PFS versus hazard ratio for survival.

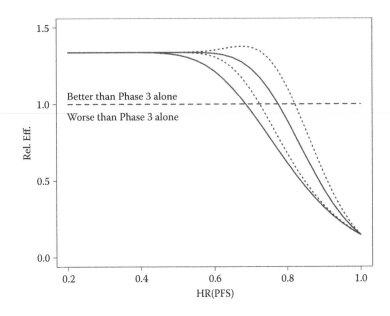

FIGURE 6.3
Relative efficiency. PFS as a surrogate for OS.

trial with survival as the primary endpoint. Thus, in the circumstances described by Figures 6.2 and 6.3, a Phase 2 screening trial with PFS as the primary endpoint can help improve the efficiency of drug development aimed at discovering clinical settings where a class of drugs may provide a survival benefit.

References

Buyse, M., Burzykowski, T., et al. 2007. Progression-free survival is a surrogate for survival in advanced colorectal cancer. *J Clin Oncol* 25(33):5218–5224.

Holmgren, E. 2008. Quantifying the usefulness of PD biomarkers in Phase 2 screening trials of oncology drugs. *Stat Med* 27(24):4928–4938.

Prentice, R.L. 1989. Surrogate endpoints in clinical trials: Definition and operational criteria. *Stat Med* 8(4):431–440.

7

Dose Selection and Subgroups:
Phase 2 as a Pilot Trial

In the previous chapters we noted there are some circumstances, particularly in the development of a new molecule, where it does not add much to the development process to use Phase 2 as a screen to see if there is sufficient activity to warrant a Phase 3 trial. In this chapter we show that a Phase 2 trial may still provide some benefit to clinical development in these circumstances when used as a pilot trial to optimize the design of a Phase 3 trial rather than as a screening trial. Using a Phase 2 trial in this way, one could ascertain whether dose strongly influences the drug's effectiveness or whether certain subsets of patients have much better responses to treatment than others.

7.1 Relative Efficiency for Selecting a Dose

Consider the problem of determining a dose to study in Phase 3. Let's evaluate a simple Phase 2/3 strategy where a control and two doses of the new molecule are studied in Phase 2 and the dose that looks the best will be studied in Phase 3. The efficiency of this strategy can be written as

$$p \cdot \frac{\left\{ \begin{matrix} \Phi\left(-\left[z_{\alpha 3} - z_\beta \right] \cdot \left(f_{\delta_1} - f_{\delta_2} \right) \cdot \sqrt{f_N \cdot \frac{2}{3}} \right) \cdot \Phi\left(z_{\alpha 3} - \left[z_{\alpha 3} - z_\beta \right] \cdot f_{\delta_1} \right) \\ + \Phi\left(-\left[z_{\alpha 3} - z_\beta \right] \cdot \left(f_{\delta_2} - f_{\delta_1} \right) \cdot \sqrt{f_N \cdot \frac{2}{3}} \right) \cdot \Phi\left(z_{\alpha 3} - \left[z_{\alpha 3} - z_\beta \right] \cdot f_{\delta_2} \right) \end{matrix} \right\}}{C + N \cdot \left(f_N + 1 \right)} \quad (7.1)$$

whereas the efficiency of a Phase 3 trial alone strategy is

$$p \cdot \frac{0.5 \cdot \Phi\left(z_{\alpha 3} - \left[z_{\alpha 3} - z_\beta \right] \cdot f_{\delta_1} \right) + 0.5 \cdot \Phi\left(z_{\alpha 3} - \left[z_{\alpha 3} - z_\beta \right] \cdot f_{\delta_2} \right)}{C + N} \quad (7.2)$$

For the efficiency of the Phase 3 trial alone strategy, we are assuming that each dose has the same chance of being selected, since they are being selected without regard to any clinical data. The relative efficiency of such a Phase 2/Phase 3 program is

$$
\frac{\left\{ \begin{array}{l} \Phi\left(-\left[z_{\alpha_3}-z_\beta\right]\cdot\left(f_{\delta_1}-f_{\delta_2}\right)\cdot\sqrt{f_N\cdot\dfrac{2}{3}}\right)\cdot\Phi\left(z_{\alpha_3}-\left[z_{\alpha_3}-z_\beta\right]\cdot f_{\delta_1}\right) \\ +\Phi\left(-\left[z_{\alpha_3}-z_\beta\right]\cdot\left(f_{\delta_2}-f_{\delta_1}\right)\cdot\sqrt{f_N\cdot\dfrac{2}{3}}\right)\cdot\Phi\left(z_{\alpha_3}-\left[z_{\alpha_3}-z_\beta\right]\cdot f_{\delta_2}\right) \end{array} \right\}}{0.5\cdot\Phi\left(z_{\alpha_3}-\left[z_{\alpha_3}-z_\beta\right]\cdot f_{\delta_1}\right)+0.5\cdot\Phi\left(z_{\alpha_3}-\left[z_{\alpha_3}-z_\beta\right]\cdot f_{\delta_2}\right)}\cdot\frac{C+N}{C+N\cdot(f_N+1)}
\tag{7.3}
$$

Here, f_{δ_1} is the treatment effect for dose 1 in terms of the proportion of the treatment effect size assumed for the Phase 3 study, f_{δ_2} is the treatment effect for dose 2, and $f_{\delta_1}-f_{\delta_2}$ is the difference in the size of the treatment effects between the two doses.

7.2 Properties of Relative Efficiency for Selecting a Dose

The relative efficiency is minimized when $f_{\delta_1}=f_{\delta_2}$ and the minimum value of the relative efficiency that is achieved is $(C + N)/(C + N \cdot [1 + f_N])$. What is more, as the difference between f_{δ_1} and f_{δ_2} increases, the relative efficiency of this Phase 2 trial increases. To see this, let's first determine the derivative of the relative efficiency with respect to f_{δ_1}.
  Let

$$
A=\Phi\left(z_{\alpha_3}-\left[z_{\alpha_3}-z_\beta\right]\cdot f_{\delta_2}\right)^2-\Phi\left(z_{\alpha_3}-\left[z_{\alpha_3}-z_\beta\right]\cdot f_{\delta_1}\right)^2
\tag{7.4}
$$

$$
B=\Phi\left(-\left[z_{\alpha_3}-z_\beta\right]\cdot\left[f_{\delta_2}-f_{\delta_1}\right]\cdot\sqrt{f_N}\right)-\Phi\left(-\left[z_{\alpha_3}-z_\beta\right]\cdot\left[f_{\delta_1}-f_{\delta_2}\right]\cdot\sqrt{f_N}\right)
\tag{7.5}
$$

and let

$$
c=(z_{\alpha_3}-z_\beta)\cdot\frac{\sqrt{f_N}}{2}<0
\tag{7.6}
$$

Then the derivative of the relative efficiency with respect to f_{δ_1} is

$$\frac{\left(\begin{array}{c} A \cdot c \cdot \dfrac{\sqrt{f_N}}{2} \cdot \phi\left(-\left[z_{\alpha_3}-z_\beta\right]\cdot\left[f_{\delta_1}-f_{\delta_2}\right]\cdot\sqrt{f_N}\right) \\ + B \cdot c \cdot \Phi\left(z_{\alpha_3}-\left[z_{\alpha_3}-z_\beta\right]\cdot f_{\delta_2}\right)\phi\left(z_{\alpha_3}-\left[z_{\alpha_3}-z_\beta\right]\cdot f_{\delta_1}\right) \end{array}\right)}{\left[0.5\cdot\Phi\left(z_{\alpha_3}-\left[z_{\alpha_3}-z_\beta\right]\cdot f_{\delta_1}\right)+0.5\cdot\Phi\left(z_{\alpha_3}-\left[z_{\alpha_3}-z_\beta\right]\cdot f_{\delta_2}\right)\right]^2} \tag{7.7}$$

When $f_{\delta_1} > f_{\delta_2}$ this derivative is positive and a reduction in f_{δ_1} decreases the relative efficiency. When $f_{\delta_1} < f_{\delta_2}$ this derivative is negative and the relative efficiency increases as f_{δ_1} decreases. A similar result can be obtained for the derivative with respect to f_{δ_2}. Thus, we see that the greater the difference between f_{δ_1} and f_{δ_2}, the greater the improvement in the relative efficiency from adding a Phase 2 pilot trial.

The magnitude of the improvement in efficiency from this use of a Phase 2 trial is illustrated in Figure 7.1. The figure presents the relative efficiency for values of f_{δ_1} ranging from 0 to 2. f_{δ_2} is assumed to equal 1 so that the treatment effect size of dose 2 relative to control is sufficient to result in 90 percent power for the Phase 3 trial.

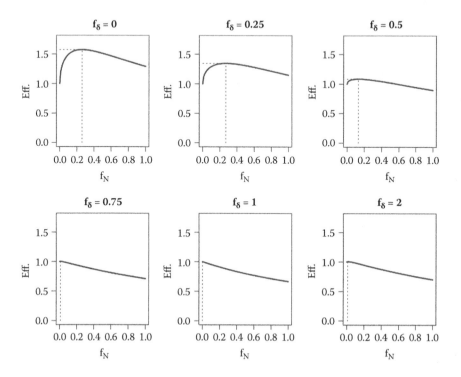

FIGURE 7.1
Relative efficiency of a pilot trial as a function of f_d and f.

For values of f_{δ_1} that are close to zero there is a large gain in efficiency over a Phase 3 trial alone strategy. That is, when one dose is not active and the other is active at the level that would make the Phase 3 trial have 90 percent power, then the gain in efficiency can be as much as 50 percent. On the other hand, there is little gain in efficiency at all when f_{δ_1} is 0.6 or more. So, when one is considering whether to do dose ranging for a drug that has achieved its target plasma concentration and is inhibiting the target, there may not be much gained from comparing two doses in Phase 2. However, if the molecule is first in class and concentrations of the drug at the target as well as inhibition of the target cannot be measured, then Phase 2 dose ranging could greatly improve the efficiency of drug development.

Figure 7.2 presents for each value of f_{δ_1} the maximum efficiency that can be attained as well as the fraction of the Phase 3 sample size f_N at which the maximum is attained. We are summing that the Phase 3 trial is a 90 percent powered study, that $C + N = 2 \cdot N$ and that $C + N \cdot (f_N + 1) = N \cdot (2 + f_N)$.

Note that the size of such a study should not be much more than 25 percent of the Phase 3 sample size. Further, as also seen in Figure 7.2, if the sample size is at least 20 percent of the Phase 3 sample size, one would be assured of achieving most of the gain in efficiency that could be attained.

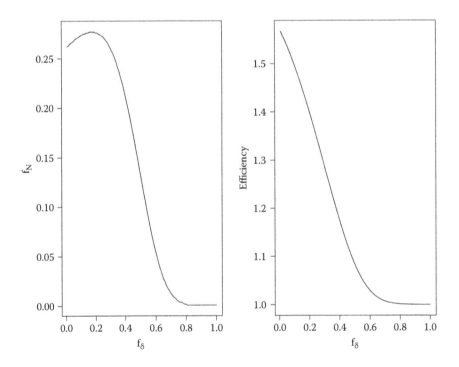

FIGURE 7.2
Maximum gain in efficiency from a Phase 2 pilot trial as a function of f.

TABLE 7.1

Relative Efficiency of a Pilot Study of Two Doses

C	f_{δ_1}	f_N 0.10	0.20	0.40	0.60	0.80	1.00
0.0	0.00	1.423	1.435	1.326	1.192	1.072	0.969
0.0	0.25	1.232	1.227	1.141	1.039	0.944	0.860
0.0	0.50	1.033	0.990	0.894	0.808	0.734	0.671
0.0	0.75	0.930	0.860	0.746	0.659	0.590	0.534
0.0	1.00	0.909	0.833	0.714	0.625	0.556	0.500
0.0	1.25	0.916	0.842	0.724	0.636	0.566	0.511
0.0	1.50	0.924	0.853	0.736	0.647	0.577	0.521
0.0	2.00	0.938	0.867	0.748	0.657	0.584	0.526
0.5	0.00	1.467	1.520	1.466	1.363	1.258	1.163
0.5	0.25	1.270	1.299	1.261	1.187	1.108	1.032
0.5	0.50	1.065	1.048	0.988	0.923	0.862	0.805
0.5	0.75	0.959	0.911	0.825	0.753	0.692	0.641
0.5	1.00	0.938	0.882	0.789	0.714	0.652	0.600
0.5	1.25	0.944	0.891	0.801	0.726	0.665	0.613
0.5	1.50	0.953	0.903	0.814	0.740	0.678	0.625
0.5	2.00	0.967	0.918	0.827	0.750	0.686	0.631
1.0	0.00	1.491	1.566	1.547	1.468	1.378	1.292
1.0	0.25	1.291	1.339	1.331	1.278	1.213	1.147
1.0	0.50	1.082	1.080	1.043	0.994	0.944	0.895
1.0	0.75	0.974	0.938	0.871	0.811	0.758	0.712
1.0	1.00	0.952	0.909	0.833	0.769	0.714	0.667
1.0	1.25	0.959	0.918	0.845	0.782	0.728	0.681
1.0	1.50	0.968	0.930	0.859	0.797	0.742	0.695
1.0	2.00	0.982	0.946	0.873	0.808	0.751	0.701

Table 7.1 provides a tabulation of the relative efficiency at various levels of C and f_{δ_1} when $f_{\delta_2} = 0$. Note that larger values of C result in larger values for efficiency. For example, when f_{δ_1} is 0.0, f_N is 0.20, and C equals 0, the relative efficiency is 1.435. However, when f_{δ_1} is 0.0, f_N is 0.20, and C equals 1, the relative efficiency is 1.566.

7.3 Relative Efficiency for Selecting a Subgroup

When one is looking for a subgroup where subjects have a good response, one is essentially asking whether the treatment effect in a subset is different from the treatment effect in its complement. Because this hypothesis involves the comparison of two treatment effects instead of the evaluation of a single treatment effect, the variability is twice what it would be in a typical Phase 3 trial. More specifically, if we let n represent the number of subjects per group in a simple two-group comparison in a Phase 3 trial and we assume all subsets have the same sample size, then we can write

$$P\left(\frac{\overline{X}_1^T - \overline{X}_1^C - \left[\overline{X}_2^T - \overline{X}_2^C\right]}{\sqrt{4 \cdot \sigma^2/(n/2)}} < z_{\alpha_3}\right) = \beta \tag{7.8}$$

$$z_{\alpha_3} - \frac{\mu_{T,1} - \mu_{C,1} - [\mu_{T,2} - \mu_{C,2}]}{\sqrt{8 \cdot \sigma^2/n}} = z_\beta \tag{7.9}$$

$$z_{\alpha_3} - z_\beta = \frac{\mu_{T,1} - \mu_{C,1} - [\mu_{T,2} - \mu_{C,2}]}{\sqrt{4 \cdot 2 \cdot \sigma^2/n}} \tag{7.10}$$

So, if the magnitude of the difference in means we are looking for is the same as with a study that simply compares two groups, that is, if

$$\mu_T - \mu_C = \mu_{T,1} - \mu_{C,1} - [\mu_{T,2} - \mu_{C,2}] \tag{7.11}$$

then the magnitude of this interaction treatment effect will be less than the treatment effect associated with a simple two-group comparison by a factor of $1/\sqrt{4}$. Consequently, the relative efficiency of a Phase 2 study designed to pick the subset with the best response to treatment can be expressed as

$$\frac{\left\{\begin{array}{l}\Phi\left(-[z_{\alpha_3} - z_\beta] \cdot \left(\dfrac{f_{\delta_1} - f_{\delta_2}}{\sqrt{4}}\right) \cdot \sqrt{f_N}\right) \cdot \Phi\left(z_{\alpha_3} - [z_{\alpha_3} - z_\beta] \cdot f_{\delta_1}\right) \\[2mm] +\Phi\left(-[z_{\alpha_3} - z_\beta] \cdot \left(\dfrac{f_{\delta_2} - f_{\delta_1}}{\sqrt{4}}\right) \cdot \sqrt{f_N}\right) \cdot \Phi\left(z_{\alpha_3} - [z_{\alpha_3} - z_\beta] \cdot f_{\delta_2}\right)\end{array}\right\}}{0.5 \cdot \Phi\left(z_{\alpha_3} - [z_{\alpha_3} - z_\beta] \cdot f_{\delta_1}\right) + 0.5 \cdot \Phi\left(z_{\alpha_3} - [z_{\alpha_3} - z_\beta] \cdot f_{\delta_2}\right)} \cdot \frac{N+C}{N+C+n} \tag{7.12}$$

The expression in Equation (7.12) is very similar to the expression for the relative efficiency for comparing two doses in Equation (7.3) except for the factor of $\sqrt{4}$ in the expressions associated with the Phase 2 study.

7.4 Evaluating the Marker Hypothesis

The "marker hypothesis" may be described as the proposition that the experimental agent has much better activity relative to subjects treated with a control among those who express a particular biologic marker at baseline. Now, if we are looking for the difference in the treatment effects between marker positive and marker negative subjects to be of roughly the same size as the magnitude of the treatment effect in a Phase 3 comparing an experimental treatment with control, then it would take a trial 4 times the size of the Phase 3 trial to definitively establish the marker hypothesis. That is, it would take a trial 4 times as big to establish that the treatment effect in the marker positive subjects is statistically different than the treatment effect in marker negative subjects. In this situation the typical Phase 3 trial may be useful as a "screening" trial for the definitive trial of the marker hypothesis. That is, since the Phase 3 trial is underpowered to definitively evaluate the marker hypothesis and because the costs of a "Stage 4" trial would be 4 times the costs of a Phase 3 trial, the Phase 3 trial is used as a screen to determine whether to do the Stage 4 trial would improve the efficiency of finding a "targeted therapy." We will explore clinical development strategies for evaluating a targeted therapy in Chapter 17.

8

Multistage Screening

Until now we have been considering how to maximize the efficiency of drug development through the optimization of the size and type 1 error of Phase 2 trials. As we mentioned at the beginning of this book, sizing a trial in one phase of drug development and then deciding whether to go on to the next phase is an issue that permeates all of drug development. In this section we adapt the approach developed for evaluating the Phase 2/3 decision problem to address the optimization of multiple screening trials that precede a definitive trial.

8.1 Efficiency

The formula we developed in Chapter 3 for the efficiency of a Phase 2/3 design is

$$\frac{p \cdot \Phi\left(z_{\alpha_2} - \left[z_{\alpha_3} - z_\beta\right] \cdot f_\delta \cdot \sqrt{f_N}\right) \cdot \Phi\left(z_{\alpha_3} - \left[z_{\alpha_3} - z_\beta\right] \cdot f_\delta\right)}{N \cdot \left[f_N + p \cdot \Phi\left(z_{\alpha_2} - \left[z_{\alpha_3} - z_\beta\right] \cdot f_\delta \cdot \sqrt{f_N}\right) + (1-p) \cdot \alpha_2\right]} \tag{8.1}$$

Adopting some new notation to facilitate the generalization to multiple studies, we may write this as

$$\frac{p \cdot Pw_2 \cdot Pw_3}{N \cdot \left[f_N + P(2 \to 3)\right]} \tag{8.2}$$

where
   Pw_2 = the power of the Phase 2 trial
   Pw_3 = the power of the Phase 3 trial
   $P(2 \to 3)$ = the probability of moving ahead from Phase 2 to Phase 3

Generalizing expression (8.2) to a series of $K-1$ independent studies, which are followed by the definitive Phase 2/3 clinical program, the efficiency can be written as

$$\frac{\displaystyle\prod_{i=1}^{K} p_i \cdot Pw_i}{N \cdot \left[f_{N,1} + \displaystyle\sum_{i=1}^{K-1} f_{N,i+1} \cdot \prod_{j=1}^{i} P(j \to j+1) \right]} \tag{8.3}$$

where

p_i = probability that the drug is effective in study i

Pw_i = the power of the ith study

$f_{N,i}$ = sample size for the ith study as a fraction of the sample size for the Kth study

$f_{N,K} = 1$

$P(j \to j + 1) = p_j \cdot Pw_j + (1 - p_j) \cdot \alpha_j$

The sequence of studies could start with, for example, a study of the drug's effectiveness in cell cultures, followed by an animal toxicology study, a study of animal pharmacokinetics, and then a Phase 2/3 clinical program.

The numerator in Equation (8.3) is the probability that a drug that is effective passes studies 1 through K, and the denominator is the expected sample size or the expected cost of conducting the studies in sequence. Note that p_K depends on the results of the previous $K - 1$ studies, while $p_1 \ldots p_{K-1}$ do not depend on the results of the previous studies by the assumption that they are independent.

The efficiency of a drug development program where study 1 precedes study 2, which precedes the definitive stage 3, is

$$\frac{p_1 \cdot p_2 \cdot p_3 \cdot Pw_1 \cdot Pw_2 \cdot Pw_3}{N \cdot \left\{ f_{N_1} + P(1 \to 2) \cdot \left[f_{N_2} + P(2 \to 3) \right] \right\}}$$

$$= \frac{p_3 \cdot Pw_3}{N} \frac{p_2 \cdot Pw_2}{f_{N_2} + P(2 \to 3)} \frac{p_1 \cdot Pw_1}{\dfrac{f_{N_1}}{f_{N_2} + P(2 \to 3)} + P(1 \to 2)} \tag{8.4}$$

The efficiency of a development program where studies 1 through 3 precede the definitive stage 4 is

$$\frac{p_1 \cdot p_2 \cdot p_3 \cdot p_4 \cdot Pw_1 \cdot Pw_2 \cdot Pw_3 \cdot Pw_4}{N \cdot \left\{ f_{N_1} + P(1 \to 2) \cdot \left[f_{N_2} + P(2 \to 3) \cdot \left(f_{N_3} + P(3 \to 4) \right) \right] \right\}}$$

$$= \frac{p_4 \cdot Pw_4}{N} \times \frac{p_3 \cdot Pw_3}{f_{N_3} + P(3 \to 4)} \times \frac{p_2 \cdot Pw_2}{\dfrac{f_{N_2}}{f_{N_3} + P(3 \to 4)} + P(2 \to 3)} \tag{8.5}$$

$$\times \frac{p_1 \cdot Pw_1}{\dfrac{f_{N_1}}{f_{N_2} + P(2 \to 3) \cdot \left(f_{N_3} + P(3 \to 4) \right)} + P(1 \to 2)}$$

In general the efficiency for a series of independent studies can be expressed as the product of the efficiencies of each study where the efficiency of a study is $A/(B + C)$ where

A = power of the study to detect a signal and move on to the next stage

B = study sample size as a fraction of the expected sample size starting with the next stage

C = probability of moving to the next stage

Note that the constant B associated with study i is a function of the treatment effect size, the type 1 error, and the sample size for each following study since they all affect the expected sample size following stage i. Further note that the larger the expected sample size following study i, the smaller B is and the greater the factor associated with study i.

8.2 Order of Tests in Drug Development

Now we address the question of what is the optimal order in which to conduct a sequence of $K - 1$ independent studies, which are followed by stage K, the Phase 2/3 clinical trial program. The efficiency of these studies ordered in sequence from $i = 1 \ldots K$ is

$$\frac{p_1 \cdot p_2 \ldots p_K \cdot Pw_1 \cdot Pw_2 \ldots \cdot Pw_K}{N\left[f_{N_1} + P(1 \to 2) \cdot f_{N_2} + \ldots + P(1 \to K-1) \cdot f_{N_{K-1}} + P(1 \to K) \cdot f_{N_K} \right]} \tag{8.6}$$

$$= \frac{p_K \cdot Pw_K}{N} \times \frac{p_1 \cdot p_2 \ldots p_{K-1} \cdot Pw_1 \cdot Pw_2 \ldots \cdot Pw_{K-1}}{f_{N_1} + P(1 \to 2) \cdot f_{N_2} + \ldots + P(1 \to K-1) \cdot f_{N_{K-1}} + P(1 \to K) \cdot f_{N_K}} \tag{8.7}$$

Note that the numerator of the second term in expression (8.7) is the same regardless of the order of the tests. The only part of this expression that depends on the order of the studies is the denominator of the second term in the product. This can be viewed as the expected cumulative cost of performing studies 1 to $K - 1$ in the order specified.

By the independence of studies $1 \ldots K - 1$, we can write the second term equivalently as

$$\frac{p_1 \cdot p_2 \cdot \ldots \cdot p_{K-1} \cdot Pw_1 \cdot Pw_2 \cdot \ldots \cdot Pw_{k-1} / P(1 \to K)}{\dfrac{f_{N_1}}{P(1 \to 2) \cdot P(2 \to 3) \cdot \ldots \cdot P(K-1 \to K)} + \dfrac{f_{N_2}}{P(2 \to 3) \cdot \ldots \cdot P(K-1 \to K)} + \ldots + f_{N_K}} \tag{8.8}$$

Now suppose that study i and study j are undertaken successively, with study j following study i. Then all that changes in the denominator of Equation (8.8) when we change the order of i and j are the terms with f_{N_i} and f_{N_j} in the numerator. Maximizing efficiency with respect to the order of study i and study j means minimizing the sum of these two terms. That is, undertaking study i before study j will maximize the efficiency if

$$\frac{f_{N_i}}{C \cdot P(i \to j) \cdot P(j \to k)} + \frac{f_{N_j}}{C \cdot P(j \to k)} < \frac{f_{N_j}}{C \cdot P(j \to i) \cdot P(i \to k)} + \frac{f_{N_i}}{C \cdot P(i \to k)} \qquad (8.9)$$

where study k immediately follows studies i and j. Since $P(i \to j) \cdot P(j \to k) = P(j \to i) \cdot P(i \to k)$ by independence, Equation (8.9) implies

$$f_{N_i} + f_{N_j} \cdot P(i \to j) < f_{N_j} + f_{N_i} \cdot P(j \to i) \qquad (8.10)$$

or

$$\frac{f_{N_i}}{f_{N_j}} < \frac{1 - P(i \to j)}{1 - P(j \to i)} \qquad (8.11)$$

Inequality (8.11) can serve as the basis of an algorithm for maximizing efficiency with respect to the order of $K - 1$ studies. If the efficiency of the whole series of studies is maximized then (8.11) must be satisfied for each pair of successive studies, which will determine a unique order for the tests. Thus, a whole series of independent studies can be evaluated in a pairwise fashion as above to determine the order that maximizes the efficiency of development.

If all of the tests have the same probability of moving to the next stage, that is, $P(i \to i + 1)$ is the same for all i, then the efficiency is maximized (cost minimized) by arranging the tests so that the corresponding costs are in increasing order, that is, so that the least expensive trials are performed before the more expensive trials. If all tests have the same cost, $f_{N_1} = f_{N_2} = \ldots = f_{N_K}$, then the tests should be arranged so that the tests with the smallest chance of moving the drug forward are performed before tests with a larger chance.

Finally, as an example, note that if the probability of passing stage i is 0.90 and the probability of passing stage j is 0.80, then test i should be performed before stage j if

$$\frac{f_{N_i}}{f_{N_j}} < \frac{1 - 0.90}{1 - 0.80} = \frac{0.10}{0.20} = 0.5 \qquad (8.12)$$

that is, if the cost of stage i is not more than half the cost of stage j.

8.3 Adverse Events

In each study that is part of a clinical program to gain marketing approval of a new molecule, the safety of the drug in patients is evaluated as well as efficacy. Adverse events are thus evaluated in multiple stages as a part of every clinical program for a new molecule. To assess the efficiency of a clinical program to detect an adverse event safety signal, we have to modify the formula developed for efficacy. Instead of continuing development at each stage if the study detects an efficacy signal, we stop development if a study detects an adverse event/safety signal at any stage. Thus, the efficiency for identifying an unsafe drug in a clinical program comprised of K studies conducted in order 1, ..., K is

$$
\frac{\pi \times \left(1 - \prod_{i=1}^{K} Pw_i\right)}{N \cdot \left[f_{N,1} + \sum_{i=1}^{K-1} f_{N,i+1} \cdot \prod_{j=1}^{i} P(j \to j+1) \right]}
\tag{8.13}
$$

where

$$
Pw_i = (1-p)^{n_i}
\tag{8.14}
$$

$$
P(j \to j+1) = \pi \cdot Pw_i + 1 - \pi
\tag{8.15}
$$

and

π = probability of a safety signal
p = incidence of safety signal in study population
n_j = number of subjects exposed to study drug

In the case of two studies where study 2 follows study 1, the efficiency for identifying a safety signal is

$$
\frac{\pi \cdot \left[1 - (1-p)^{n_1} \cdot (1-p)^{n_2}\right]}{n_2 \cdot \left(f_{N,1} + f_{N,2} \cdot \left[\pi \cdot (1-p)^{n_1} + 1 - \pi\right]\right)}
\tag{8.16}
$$

$$
= \frac{\pi \cdot \left[1 - (1-p)^{n_2}\right]}{n_2} \cdot \frac{\dfrac{1 - (1-p)^{n_1+n_2}}{1 - (1-p)^{n_2}}}{f_{N,1} + f_{N,2} \cdot \left[\pi \cdot (1-p)^{n_1} + 1 - \pi\right]}
$$

Note that $f_{N,2} = 1$. The first term on the right of Equation (8.16) is the efficiency of a single study with n_2 subjects. The second term in the product on the right-hand side is once again the relative efficiency. Notice that the limit of the relative efficiency as p goes to zero is one.

$$\lim_{p \to 0} \frac{\dfrac{1-(1-p)^{n_1+n_2}}{1-(1-p)^{n_2}}}{f_{N,1}+1 \cdot \left[\pi \cdot (1-p)^{n_1} + 1 - \pi\right]} = \lim_{p \to 0} \frac{\dfrac{-(n_1+n_2) \cdot (1-p)^{n_1+n_2-1}}{-n_2 \cdot (1-p)^{n_2-1}}}{f_{N,1}+1} \tag{8.17}$$

$$= \frac{\dfrac{n_1+n_2}{n_2}}{\dfrac{n_1}{n_2}+1} = 1 \tag{8.18}$$

The limit as p goes to one is

$$\frac{1}{n_1/n_2+1-\pi} \tag{8.19}$$

So, if $n_1/n_2 + 1 - \pi$ is small enough, the relative efficiency of determining the drug is not safe will be greater than 1 for a range of values for p.

We can express the relative efficiency as

$$\frac{\dfrac{1-(1-p)^{n_1+n_2}}{\left[f_{N,2} \cdot \pi \cdot (1-p)^{n_1} + a\right] \cdot \left[1-(1-p)^{n_2}\right]}}{}$$

$$= \frac{1-(1-p)^{n_1+n_2}}{a - f_{N,2} \cdot \pi (1-p)^{n_1+n_2} + f_{N,2} \cdot \pi (1-p)^{n_1} - a(1-p)^{n_2}} \tag{8.20}$$

where

$$a = \frac{n_1}{n_2} + f_{N_2} \cdot (1-\pi) \tag{8.21}$$

In this situation with just two studies $f_{N_2} = 1$. The expression in (8.20) for the relative efficiency shows that the convergence to $1/a$ as $p \to 1$ is rather fast. The greater n_1 and n_2 the faster the convergence.

Typically, a clinical program consists of three stages starting with the Phase 1 first-in-man trial followed by a Phase 2 trial looking for signs of activity and ending with the Phase 3 confirmatory trial. The expression for the efficiency of evaluating safety in these three studies is

$$\frac{\pi \cdot \left[1-(1-p)^N\right]}{N} \times \frac{\dfrac{1-(1-p)^{N(1+f_{N2})}}{1-(1-p)^N}}{f_{N_2} + P(2 \to 3)} \times \frac{\dfrac{1-(1-p)^{N(1+f_{N2}+f_{N1})}}{1-(1-p)^{N(1+f_{N2})}}}{\dfrac{f_{N_1}}{f_{N_2} + P(2 \to 3)} + P(1 \to 2)} \tag{8.22}$$

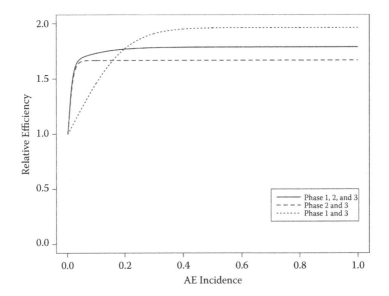

FIGURE 8.1
Relative efficiency of identifying a safety signal.

The numerator in the second and third terms represents the factor by which the probability of detecting the safety signal changes when the stage is added. Figure 8.1 displays the relative efficiency of a Phase 1 trial prior to a Phase 3, a Phase 2 trial prior to a Phase 3, and Phase 1 and Phase 2 trial prior to a Phase 3 trial. Note that the efficiency of a program that includes Phases 1, 2, and 3 is better than a program that includes only Phases 2 and 3, especially for safety signals with an incidence greater than 5 percent. For detecting safety signals with a high incidence, a clinical program where a Phase 1 trial is followed by a Phase 3 trial would be the most efficient. However, this program would not be as efficient as the others for detecting a safety signal with an incidence less than 20 percent.

Section II

A Theory of Evidence in Drug Development

9

Preference for Simple Tests of Hypotheses over Model-Based Tests

This chapter begins an exploration of three important properties that impact the strength of evidence developed by a clinical trial program to support marketing approval of a new drug: the supporting statistical test, the determination of what is a "positive" result, and the degree of confirmation. This chapter will explore the statistical test and in particular the preference for simple tests of hypotheses over model-based tests. Chapter 10 will consider how to determine when a study is positive based on the power and type 1 error of the specified statistical test. Chapter 11 addresses confirmation and looks at evidence developed in a Phase 2/3 clinical program from the perspective of a reviewer of positive trials that are submitted with applications for marketing approval. These three chapters together comprise a theory of evidence in drug development.

In the evaluation of clinical trial data, regulators generally prefer simple hypothesis tests over model-based tests to determine whether a drug is effective. For example, in the evaluation of a drug that reduces blood pressure, a Z-test based on the difference between the test treatment and control of the mean change in systolic blood pressure from baseline where the important baseline factors are balanced between treatment groups would be preferred over a test based on a linear model of the change in systolic blood pressure that includes a term for treatment along with terms for other baseline variables that are imbalanced between the arms of the study. The underlying reason for this is that the model-based test is dependent on more estimates of related parameters than is the simple difference in means and thus requires more assumptions to be correct. In what follows we will look at the variance of a model-based estimate of the treatment effect that accounts for baseline variables that are imbalanced between the arms of the study and compare it with the variance of a simple difference in means to help understand why there is a preference for simple hypothesis tests.

9.1 Control Maximum Risk

First, we want to take note of a principle that underlies all three chapters concerned with the strength of evidence from a drug development program. Regulators are gatekeepers set up by society to make sure that drugs sold to the public are truly effective. It is therefore up to the sponsors of a new drug to convince regulators that their drug is effective. As such, test procedures that maximize the minimum power and are calibrated within a study design so as to set the minimum power among all treatment effects of interest at an acceptable level provide the best evidence of a drug's activity since regardless of the true state of nature the risk borne by society and the regulators if the drug is approved is at an acceptable level.

9.2 Variance of a Model-Based Estimate of Treatment Effect

To begin an examination of the variance of a model-based estimate of the treatment effect, let's suppose that subjects are randomized to two groups—a control group and an experimental treatment group—and that the changes in their systolic blood pressure from baseline are represented as $Y_{C,1}, ..., Y_{C,N}$ and $Y_{T,1}, ..., Y_{T,N}$. Let $X_{C,1}, ..., X_{C,N}$ and $X_{T,1}, ..., X_{T,N}$ represent a baseline covariate that is measured on each patient in the treatment and control arm, and consider the following model

$$Y = \beta_0 + \beta_1 \cdot I_{Trt} + \beta_2 \cdot X + \varepsilon \tag{9.1}$$

where I_{Trt} is an indicator variable that marks subjects who received the experimental treatment. In this equation, β_1 represents the effect on Y provided by the experimental treatment over and above control.

We can write this equation in matrix form as

$$Y = X \cdot \beta + \varepsilon \tag{9.2}$$

where $\varepsilon \sim N(0, \sigma_\varepsilon^2)$. The well known least squares solution for β is

$$\beta = (X'X)^{-1} X'Y \tag{9.3}$$

and the variance of β is

$$(X'X)^{-1} \sigma_\varepsilon^2 \tag{9.4}$$

We are particularly interested in the coefficient of the model that represents the magnitude of the treatment effect. The variance for this term can be found in the second row and second column of the variance covariance matrix for the coefficients in the model. The matrix, $X'X$, can be represented in more detail as

$$
X'X = \begin{bmatrix}
N_C + N_T & N_T & \sum X_C + \sum X_T \\
N_T & N_T & \sum X_T \\
\sum X_C + \sum X_T & \sum X_T & \sum X_C^2 + \sum X_T^2
\end{bmatrix}
\tag{9.5}
$$

Using the determinant form of the inverse we can write the variance for the estimate of the treatment effect as

$$
\frac{\begin{vmatrix}
N_C + N_T & \sum X_C + \sum X_T \\
\sum X_C + \sum X_T & \sum X_C^2 + \sum X_T^2
\end{vmatrix}}{\begin{vmatrix}
N_C + N_T & N_T & \sum X_C + \sum X_T \\
N_T & N_T & \sum X_T \\
\sum X_C + \sum X_T & \sum X_T & \sum X_C^2 + \sum X_T^2
\end{vmatrix}} \cdot \sigma_\varepsilon^2
\tag{9.6}
$$

$$
= \frac{(N_C + N_T) \cdot \left(\sum X_C^2 + \sum X_T^2\right) - \left(\sum X_C + \sum X_T\right)^2}{A + B + C} \cdot \left(1 - R^2\right) \cdot \sigma_y^2
\tag{9.7}
$$

where

$$
A = (N_C + N_T)\left[N_T \cdot \left(\sum X_C^2 + \sum X_T^2\right) - \left(\sum X_T\right)^2 \right]
\tag{9.8}
$$

$$
B = -N_T\left[N_T \cdot \left(\sum X_C^2 + \sum X_T^2\right) - \left(\sum X_C + \sum X_T\right) \cdot \sum X_T \right]
\tag{9.9}
$$

$$
C = \left(\sum X_C + \sum X_T\right)\left[N_T \left(\sum X_T\right) - \left(\sum X_C + \sum X_T\right) \cdot N_T \right]
\tag{9.10}
$$

With some algebra, (9.7) reduces to

$$
\left(\frac{1}{N_C} + \frac{1}{N_T}\right) \cdot \frac{\left[\left(\sum X_C^2 + \sum X_T^2\right) - \dfrac{\left(\sum X_C + \sum X_T\right)^2}{N_C + N_T}\right]}{\left[\sum X_C^2 - \dfrac{\left(\sum X_C\right)^2}{N_C} + \sum X_T^2 - \dfrac{\left(\sum X_T\right)^2}{N_T}\right]} \cdot \left(1 - R^2\right) \cdot \sigma_y^2
\tag{9.11}
$$

$$= \left(\frac{1}{N_C} + \frac{1}{N_T} \right) \cdot \left[\frac{(N_C + N_T)\,\text{var}(X)}{N_C \cdot \text{var}(X_C) + N_T \cdot \text{var}(X_T)} \right] \cdot \left(1 - R^2 \right) \cdot \sigma_y^2 \qquad (9.12)$$

$$= \left(\frac{1}{N_C} + \frac{1}{N_T} \right) \cdot \left[\frac{\left\{ N_C \cdot \text{var}(X_C) + N_T \cdot \text{var}(X_T) + \dfrac{N_C \cdot N_T}{N_C + N_T} \left(\bar{X}_C - \bar{X}_T \right)^2 \right\}}{N_C \cdot \text{var}(X_C) + N_T \cdot \text{var}(X_T)} \right] \qquad (9.13)$$

$$\cdot \left(1 - R^2 \right) \cdot \sigma_y^2$$

It can be seen from Equation (9.13) that the greater the imbalance between $\bar{X}_C$ and $\bar{X}_T$ the greater the variability in the estimate of the treatment effect, assuming of course that $(1 - R^2) \cdot \sigma_y^2$ does not change. Note that the variance inflation resulting from the imbalance between $\bar{X}_C$ and $\bar{X}_T$ does not depend on the scale of measurement. That is, if the scale of measurement changes by a factor of k, then the square of the difference in the sample means will increase by a factor of k^2 as will $\text{var}(X_C)$ and $\text{var}(X_T)$.

The estimate of β involves the other two terms in the second row of $(X'X)^{-1}$ and can thus be expressed as

$$\beta = -A_1 \cdot \left(\sum Y_T + \sum Y_C \right) + A_2 \cdot \left(\sum Y_T \right) - A_3 \cdot \left(\sum X_T \cdot Y_T + \sum X_C \cdot Y_C \right) \quad (9.14)$$

where

$$A_1 = \frac{N_T \cdot \left(\sum X_C^2 + \sum X_T^2 \right) - \left(\sum X_T \right) \left(\sum X_C + \sum X_T \right)}{A + B + C}$$

$$= \frac{(N_T + N_C) N_T \left[\dfrac{\sum X_C^2 + \sum X_T^2}{N_T + N_C} - \dfrac{\sum X_T}{N_T} \dfrac{\left(\sum X_C + \sum X_T \right)}{N_T + N_C} \right]}{N_T N_C \left(N_C\, \text{var}(X_C) + N_T\, \text{var}(X_T) \right)} \qquad (9.15)$$

$$A_2 = \frac{(N_T + N_C) \cdot (N_T + N_C) \cdot \left[\dfrac{\sum X_C^2 + \sum X_T^2}{N_T + N_C} - \dfrac{\left(\sum X_C + \sum X_T \right)^2}{(N_T + N_C)^2} \right]}{N_T N_C \left(N_C\, \text{var}(X_C) + N_T\, \text{var}(X_T) \right)} \qquad (9.16)$$

$$A_3 = \frac{(N_C + N_T) \cdot \left(\sum X_T \right) - \left(\sum X_C + \sum X_T \right) \cdot N_T}{A + B + C} \qquad (9.17)$$

$$= \frac{N_C \sum X_T - N_T \sum X_C}{N_T N_C \left(N_C \, \mathrm{var}(X_C) + N_T \, \mathrm{var}(X_T) \right)} \tag{9.18}$$

Note that when the randomization to the control arm and the treatment arm is effective in balancing the two arms, and an equal number of subjects are allocated to the two arms we have that

$$A_1 = \frac{2 \cdot N^2 \cdot \mathrm{var}(X)}{N^3 \cdot 2 \cdot \mathrm{var}(X)} = \frac{1}{N} \tag{9.19}$$

$$A_2 = \frac{4 \cdot N^2 \cdot \mathrm{var}(X)}{2 \cdot N^3 \cdot \mathrm{var}(X)} = \frac{2}{N} \tag{9.20}$$

$$A_3 = \frac{N^2 \cdot (E(X) - E(X))}{N^3 \cdot 2 \cdot \mathrm{var}(X)} = 0 \tag{9.21}$$

and so the estimate is approximately

$$\frac{-1}{N} \cdot \left(\sum Y_T + \sum Y_C \right) + \frac{2}{N} \sum Y_T = \frac{\sum Y_T}{N} - \frac{\sum Y_C}{N} \tag{9.22}$$

When

$$\frac{\sum X_T}{N_T} > \frac{\sum X_C + \sum X_T}{N_C + N_T} \tag{9.23}$$

A_1 will be smaller than in the balanced case and so the estimate of the treatment effect will move closer to $\sum Y_T$. On the other hand, if

$$\frac{\sum X_T}{N_T} < \frac{\sum X_C + \sum X_T}{N_C + N_T} \tag{9.24}$$

then A_1 will be larger than in the balanced case and the estimate of the treatment effect will move closer to

$$-1 \cdot \left(\sum Y_T + \sum Y_C \right) \tag{9.25}$$

The impact of imbalances on A_2 and A_3 must also be considered to gauge the complete impact of an imbalance in X on the estimate of the treatment effect.

9.3 Comparison of a Simple Difference in Means with a Model-Based Estimate of Treatment Effect

Figure 9.1 presents the variance of the estimate of the treatment effect as a function of the imbalance in X and the correlation between X and Y for both the simple difference in means and the model adjusted estimate as described

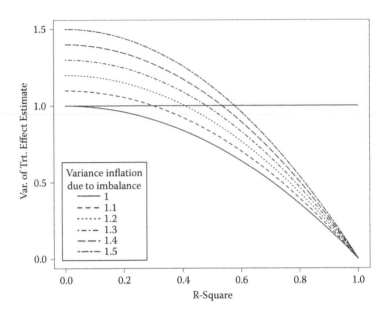

FIGURE 9.1
Variance of a model-based estimate of treatment effect as a function of the correlation and imbalance in an associated covariate.

in Equation (9.13). The solid horizontal line represents the variance of the simple difference in means, $\bar{Y}_T - \bar{Y}_C$, in the sample space of all possible outcomes of the experiment. It is a horizontal line because it does not depend on the correlation between X and Y, nor does it depend on the imbalance between $\bar{X}_C$ and $\bar{X}_T$. In contrast, the variance of the estimate from the linear model, in the sample space where there is a specific imbalance in the covariate X, is always greater than one for some range of values for the correlation that includes zero.

It is difficult to compare the power of the simple difference in means with the model-based estimate of the treatment effect when the variance is calculated for different sample spaces as in Figure 9.1. We will now formally compare the power of the simple difference in means with the power for the model-based estimate of the treatment effect averaged over the whole sample space when the covariates included in the model are those with an imbalance between the treatment arms.

As before, suppose that the variable of interest is Y and that we have collected the data $Y_{C,1} \ldots Y_{C,n}$ and $Y_{T,1} \ldots Y_{T,n}$ from a randomized trial where $Y_C \sim N(0, \sigma^2)$ and $Y_T \sim N(\delta, \sigma^2)$ so that the treatment effect is represented by the parameter δ. Suppose that there are K covariates of interest. For $i = 1, \ldots, K$ let $E(Cov_{i,T})$ and $E(Cov_{i,C})$ represent the mean of covariate i in the treatment and control arms respectively, $Imb_i = \left| E\left(Cov_{i,T}\right) - E\left(Cov_{i,C}\right)\right|$, and define A_i, a subset of the sample space, as

$$A_i = \{\omega \in \Omega : \mathrm{Imb}_i > \varepsilon\} \qquad (9.26)$$

Further define

$$A_{K+1} = \left[\bigcup_{i=1}^{K} A_i \right]^c \qquad (9.27)$$

All K covariates are balanced in the set A_{K+1}. For each $\omega \in \Omega$ construct the following model

$$y = \beta_0 + \beta_{Trt} \cdot I_{Trt} + \sum_{i=1}^{K} \beta_{Cov_i} \cdot Cov_i \cdot I_{\mathrm{Imb}_i > \eta} \qquad (9.28)$$

The parameter β_{Trt} represents the model-based estimate of the treatment effect. Only those covariates with an imbalance greater than η are included in the linear model. Across the whole sample space there are only a finite number of unique models and the collection of unique models induces a partition, $\{B_j\}$, on the sample space Ω. Assume that the errors for the regression model are conditionally independent of the covariates. Then, the power of the model-based analysis is

$$\sum_j \int_{B_j} P\left(\frac{Estimate_{model}}{\sqrt{Var_{model}}} > z_{1-\alpha} \mid \mathrm{Imb}_1 = \eta_1 \ldots \mathrm{Imb}_K = \eta_K \right)$$

$$\cdot f_{\mathrm{Imb}_1,\ldots,\mathrm{Imb}_K}(\eta_1 \ldots \eta_K) \cdot d\eta_1 \cdot \ldots \cdot d\eta_K \qquad (9.29)$$

$$= \sum_j \int_{B_j} P\left(Z > z_{1-\alpha} - \frac{\delta}{\sqrt{Var_{model|\mathrm{Imb}_1=\eta_1 \ldots \mathrm{Imb}_K=\eta_K}}} \right)$$

$$\cdot f_{\mathrm{Imb}_1,\ldots,\mathrm{Imb}_K}(\eta_1 \ldots \eta_K) \cdot d\eta_1 \cdot \ldots \cdot d\eta_K \qquad (9.30)$$

The equation follows since the data are from a randomized experiment and the model-based estimate is an unbiased estimate of δ given any sort of imbalance between the treatment arms. Since the study is randomized, imbalances in unknown covariates are accounted for in the variability of the treatment effect estimate. Now we can continue the series of equations as

$$\sum_j \int_{B_j} P\left(Z > z_{1-\alpha} - \frac{\delta}{\sqrt{Var_{model|\mathrm{Imb}_1=\eta_1 \ldots \mathrm{Imb}_K=\eta_K}}} \right)$$

$$\cdot f_{\mathrm{Imb}_1,\ldots,\mathrm{Imb}_K}(\eta_1 \ldots \eta_K) \cdot d\eta_1 \cdot \ldots \cdot d\eta_K \qquad (9.31)$$

$$< \sum_j \int_{B_j} P\left(Z > z_{1-\alpha} - \frac{\delta}{\sqrt{2 \cdot \sigma^2/n}} \right) \cdot f_{\text{Imb}_1, \ldots, \text{Imb}_K}\left(\eta_1 \ldots \eta_K \right) \cdot d\eta_1 \cdot \ldots \cdot d\eta_K \qquad (9.32)$$

$$= P\left(Z > z_{1-\alpha} - \frac{\delta}{\sqrt{2 \cdot \sigma^2/n}} \right) \qquad (9.33)$$

These equations follow since the variance for the difference in means is less than the variance of the model-based estimate of the treatment effect conditioned on the imbalance in a covariate when R^2 is close to zero. The last term in the series of equations is the power for the simple difference in means. So we have shown that a model-based, data-driven estimate of the treatment effect will have less power than the simple difference in means when averaged over the whole sample space under the assumption that R^2 is small.

Suppose now that the difference in means is statistically significant and further that the randomization was effective in balancing important known prognostic factors between the two groups. Then, since the power of the test based on the difference in means is sufficient by the design of the study regardless of the true relationship with other prognostic variables, known and unknown, and since there is no need to consider adjusting the estimate of the treatment effect for imbalances in known prognostic variables, the simple difference in means provides a sound basis for granting marketing approval in these circumstances.

On the other hand, suppose that the simple difference in means is not statistically significant. Suppose further that there is an imbalance in an important prognostic variable and that after adjustment using a linear model, the treatment benefit is statistically significant. What are the risks that the regulator and society face if approval is granted in this situation? As Figure 9.1 shows, the variability in the estimate of the treatment effect depends on the true relationship between the primary endpoint and the dependent variable in the linear model as well as the observed magnitude of the imbalance. Further, we showed that the power of the model-based estimate of the treatment effect that includes covariates that are imbalanced between the arms of the study has less power than the simple difference in means when R^2 is small. When R^2 is large the power can increase quite substantially. However, the true correlation between Y and the covariates is unknown and if the true strength of the association between the primary endpoint and the covariates in the linear model is not as strong as estimated from the data, then the risk the regulator and society will be assuming will be greater than it appears from the results of the model. What's more, the risk could be greater than the risk that is assumed when the evidence in favor of a drug's approval is based on a simple difference in means that is statistically significant without any imbalances in important prognostic factors to worry about. The point here is that the exact level of risk being assumed by society is uncertain and the burden of showing the risk is acceptable falls on the sponsor of the new drug. It is not up to society to bear this additional risk; it is up to the sponsor to collect the information that is necessary to show that the risk is acceptable. In this situation, the evidence from the model-based test is not as convincing as in the case where the simple difference in means is statistically significant and not associated with imbalances in important prognostic variables. In these circumstances, it would be reasonable to ask for a follow-up trial to add strength to the evidence in support of the drug's effectiveness.

This is not to say that a simple difference in means is a better estimate of the treatment effect than the estimate from a model when there is an imbalance in a covariate that is strongly associated with the dependent variable. Indeed, the simple difference in means would be biased in this case and the model-based estimate has a chance to be unbiased. Rather, the point is that a simple difference in means when important covariates are balanced between the treatment arms is the best evidence one can obtain that the drug is effective, better than a model-based assessment that adjusts for an observed imbalance. This underlines the importance of randomization in the conduct of a study. If the randomization fails to balance important prognostic factors, then the strength of the evidence provided by the study is weakened. Hence, stratifying the randomization scheme for a study on important prognostic features or employing a dynamic randomization algorithm to assure balance across many important prognostic features helps to strengthen the evidence provided by the study ensuring that the simple difference in means will be viewed as unaffected by imbalances in other variables and consequently not requiring adjustment.

In the big picture, the burden of proving that a new molecule actually provides benefit to patients lies completely on the drug company who submits an application to the government. It is incumbent on the drug company to convince regulators that under any reasonable scenario the drug works. Thus, it is not enough to show that a p-value is less than 0.025 regardless of the test. P-values from different tests mean different things. As we saw in this chapter, a p-value from a simple comparison of means with balance in important baseline factors provides stronger evidence in favor of drug approval than a p-value for the estimate of the treatment effect in a model that contains additional baseline covariates that are imbalanced.

9.4 A Study Design That Permits Data-Driven Model Adjustment of the Treatment Effect Estimate

Now let's consider how to design a study to permit a data-driven, model-based adjustment of the treatment effect that includes baseline factors that are imbalanced between the arms of the study as covariates. The strategy will be to make sure that the power of the model-adjusted estimate is sufficient. First, let's obtain a lower bound on the power of the model adjusted estimate of the treatment effect.

Define

$$C_1 = \{\omega : \text{Imb}_i > \varepsilon_1, \text{ for no more than } L \text{ covariates}\} \qquad (9.34)$$

and

$$C_2 = \{\omega : \text{Imb}_i < \varepsilon_2, i = 1 \ldots K\} \qquad (9.35)$$

If the imbalance in a covariate is less than ε_1, the covariate will not be included in the model used to adjust the estimate of the treatment effect. ε_2 will be determined such that $P(C_2^C)$, the probability of an imbalance in any one of the K covariates, is very small. The power of the model-adjusted estimate can then be written as

$$\sum_j \int_{B_j} P\left(\frac{Estimate_{\text{model}}}{\sqrt{Var_{\text{model}}}} > z_{1-\alpha} \mid \text{Imb}_1 = \eta_1 \ldots \text{Imb}_K = \eta_K \right)$$
$$\cdot f_{\text{Imb}_1,\ldots,\text{Imb}_K}(\eta_1 \ldots \eta_K) \cdot d\eta_1 \cdot \ldots \cdot d\eta_K \qquad (9.36)$$

$$= \sum_j \int_{B_j \cap C_1 \cap C_2} P\left(\frac{Estimate_{\text{model}}}{\sqrt{Var_{\text{model}}}} > z_{1-\alpha} \mid \text{Imb}_1 = \eta_1 \ldots \text{Imb}_K = \eta_K \right)$$
$$\cdot f_{\text{Imb}_1,\ldots,\text{Imb}_K}(\eta_1 \ldots \eta_K) \cdot d\eta_1 \cdot \ldots \cdot d\eta_K$$

$$+ \sum_j \int_{B_j \cap \{C_1^c \cup C_2^c\}} P\left(\frac{Estimate_{\text{model}}}{\sqrt{Var_{\text{model}}}} > z_{1-\alpha} \mid \text{Imb}_1 = \eta_1 \ldots \text{Imb}_K = \eta_K \right) \qquad (9.37)$$
$$\cdot f_{\text{Imb}_1,\ldots,\text{Imb}_K}(\eta_1 \ldots \eta_K) \cdot d\eta_1 \cdot \ldots \cdot d\eta_K$$

$$> \sum_j \int_{B_j \cap C_1 \cap C_2} P\left(Z > z_{1-\alpha} - \frac{\delta}{\sqrt{Var_{\text{model}}}} \mid \text{Imb}_1 = \eta_1 \ldots \text{Imb}_K = \eta_K \right)$$
$$\cdot f_{\text{Imb}_1,\ldots,\text{Imb}_K}(\eta_1 \ldots \eta_K) \cdot d\eta_1 \cdot \ldots \cdot d\eta_K \qquad (9.38)$$

Now for notational purposes let $\max(Var) = Var_{\text{model} \mid L \text{ cov and Imb}=\varepsilon_2}$. $max(Var)$ represent the maximum variance inflation that can occur in $\left\{ \bigcup_j B_j \right\} \cap C_1 \cap C_2$.

Then

$$\sum_j \int_{B_j \cap C_1 \cap C_2} P\left(Z > z_{1-\alpha} - \frac{\delta}{\sqrt{Var_{model}}} \,\middle|\, Imb_1 = \eta_1 \ldots Imb_K = \eta_K \right)$$

$$\cdot f_{Imb_1, \ldots, Imb_K}\left(\eta_1 \ldots \eta_K \right) \cdot d\eta_1 \cdot \ldots \cdot d\eta_K \tag{9.39}$$

$$> P\left(Z > z_{1-\alpha} - \frac{\delta}{\sqrt{max(Var)}} \right) \cdot P\left(\begin{array}{l} \{\text{No more than } L \; \varepsilon_1 \text{ imbal. covariates}\} \\ \cap \{\text{All imbal.} \leq \varepsilon_2\} \end{array} \right) \tag{9.40}$$

$$> P\left(Z > z_{1-\alpha} - \frac{\delta}{\sqrt{max(Var)}} \right) \cdot \left[\begin{array}{l} 1 - P(> L \; \varepsilon_1 \text{ imbal. covariates}) \\ - P(\text{At least one imbal.} > \varepsilon_2) \end{array} \right] \tag{9.41}$$

The probabilities regarding imbalanced covariates in Equations (9.40) and (9.41) are calculated assuming that the differences between the treatment arms are normally distributed with mean zero. The mean zero assumption stems from the fact that the data are generated in a study where subjects are randomized to their treatment assignment.

These equations show that if a protocol includes the following elements, then the data-driven model adjustment of the estimate of treatment effect will have sufficient power. These items are

- Specify in the protocol a list of important covariates that will be looked at to assess whether an imbalance warrants a model-based covariate adjustment.

- Show that the probability of seeing more than L covariates in the list with an imbalance greater than ε_1 is close to zero. ε_1 becomes the threshold for how large an imbalance must be in order for it to be included in a model for adjusting the treatment effect estimate.

- Show that the probability of at least one covariate in the list with an imbalance greater than ε_2 is small.

- Increase the sample size of the trial above what would be sufficient for a simple test based on the difference in the mean changes from baseline to offset the loss of power due to the potential variance inflation from adjusting the treatment effect estimate for an imbalanced covariate.

Now let's consider an example to see how large the sample size adjustment may need to be in order to support a data-driven, model-based adjustment to the treatment effect estimate. Suppose we have a randomized study with 400 subjects per arm and that 10 covariates are potentially important to include in a

TABLE 9.1

Probabilities of Observing Imbalanced Covariates

Number of Subjects per Group	Number of Covariates	Imbalance as a Fraction of SD of Cov (x)	P (Imbalance > x)	Probability at Least 1 Covariate Imbalanced*	Probability More Than 3 Covariates Imbalanced > x*
400	10	0.10	0.157	0.819	0.058
400	10	0.11	0.120	0.721	0.024
400	*10*	*0.12*	0.090	0.609	*0.009*
400	10	0.13	0.066	0.495	0.003
400	10	0.14	0.048	0.387	0.001
400	10	0.15	0.034	0.292	0.000
400	10	0.16	0.024	0.213	0.000
400	10	0.17	0.016	0.151	0.000
400	10	0.18	0.011	0.104	0.000
400	10	0.19	0.007	0.070	0.000
400	10	0.20	0.005	0.046	0.000
400	10	0.21	0.003	0.029	0.000
400	10	0.22	0.002	0.018	0.000
400	10	0.23	0.001	0.011	0.000
400	*10*	*0.24*	0.001	*0.007*	0.000

* Probability is calculated assuming that the covariates are independent.

model if they happened to be imbalanced between the treatment arms. Table 9.1 presents the probability of observing imbalances of various magnitudes.

To continue this example, we will take $L = 3$ and will require that an imbalance in a covariate be more than 12 percent of its standard deviation before it will be included in a model to adjust the estimate of the treatment effect. So, for example, if gender is on the list of covariates to be considered for inclusion in the model and half the study subjects are women, then an imbalance of more than $\sqrt{0.50^2 \cdot 0.12} = 0.06$, or 6 percent, in the proportion of subjects who are women would lead to gender being included in the model. We will also take ε_2 to be 0.24. When we substitute the numbers from Table 9.1 into Equation (9.41) we have

$$P\left(Z > z_{1-\alpha} - \frac{\delta}{\sqrt{\max(Var)}}\right) \cdot [1 - 0.009 - 0.007] \qquad (9.42)$$

The final number we need to compute the sample size adjustment is the variance inflation resulting from three covariates with an imbalance of 0.24. We determined this from a simulation with 300,000 replications under the assumption that the covariates are independent and found it to equal 9.47 percent. So, the sample size must increase 9.47 percent to offset the variance inflation. We also lost $0.80(0.009 + 0.007) = 0.0128$ of the power when creating the bound. To compensate for this drop in power of 1.6 percent ($0.0128/0.80$) we need to increase the sample size by 3.4 percent. The 3.4 percent increase in sample size was calculated as indicated in Equations (9.43) through (9.45):

$$0.80 = \Phi\left(z_\alpha - \delta\sqrt{n}\right) \tag{9.43}$$

$$0.80 \times 1.016 = \Phi\left(z_\alpha + [z_{0.80} - z_\alpha] \cdot \sqrt{f_n}\right) \tag{9.44}$$

$$f_n = \left(\frac{z_{0.80 \times 1.016} - z_\alpha}{z_{0.80} - z_\alpha}\right)^2 = 1.0336 \tag{9.45}$$

So in total, the sample size needs to increase by a factor of $1.0947 \times 1.0336 = 1.131$, or roughly 13 percent, in order to offset the loss in power from the variance inflation arising from the model-adjusted estimate of the treatment effect. A test based on the model adjusted estimate of the treatment effect in these circumstances should carry the same weight as an appropriately powered test based on the simple difference in the mean changes from baseline. It should be noted that the lower bound for the power developed earlier may be improved upon. Such improvements in the lower bound will lead to smaller increases in the sample required to offset the loss of power.

10

Quantifying the Strength of
Evidence from a Study

The ultimate aim of government agencies that regulate the marketing of new drugs is to ensure that the drugs that are available for people to use are safe and effective. However, regardless of how the decision to grant marketing approval is made, there will always be some drugs that are approved that are not effective. A measure of the quality of the decision rule for granting marketing approval should therefore compare in some way the number of drugs that are approved and effective relative to those that are approved and are ineffective. One such measure is the ratio of true positives to false positives. In this chapter, we develop the ratio of true to false positives and the ratio of power to type 1 error as measures of the strength of evidence in the design and evaluation of clinical trials.

10.1 Ratio of True Positives to False Positives

A natural measure by which to gauge whether the number of ineffective drugs receiving approval is sufficiently small is the ratio of the number of effective drugs to the number of ineffective drugs that are approved. The greater this ratio the better the drug development process is at producing effective drugs for patients. In probabilistic terms, we can describe this measure of the quality of the drug development process as the ratio of the probability of a true positive to the probability of a false positive, which will be represented by the expression $P(+, T)/P(+, F)$. The plus sign (+) indicates that the study result is positive, and T and F indicate, respectively, that the drug is truly effective or ineffective.

10.1.1 Societal Benefit

One can show in a simple model that $P(+, T)/P(+, F)$ is key to determining whether society benefits from an approval decision and that the ratio of power to type 1 error, β/α, is the key element of a study design that influences the net societal benefit from a drug approval. To that end suppose that there are two states of nature. In state 0 the drug under consideration is not effective, whereas in state 1 the drug is effective with a treatment benefit represented by θ. The probability of these states of nature occurring are, respectively, p_0 and p_1, where $p_0 + p_1 = 1$. α and β are controlled by the experimenter, and p_0 and p_1 reflect the quality of the basic science underlying the selection of drug candidates for clinical development. Note that this is also the model we used to evaluate the efficiency of drug development. Further, let A represent the benefit to society from an approved drug that is truly effective and B represent the costs to society from an approved drug that is not effective. We introduce A and B to help identify the form of the statistical evidence that is required to support drug approval. It is not intended that A and B be determined for every drug project. Finally, let i index studies. Then, the net benefit to society from drugs receiving approval can be represented as

$$\sum_i \left[P(+, T) \cdot A_i - P(+, F) \cdot B_i \right] = P(+, F) \cdot \sum_i \left[\frac{P(+, T)}{P(+, F)} \cdot A_i - B_i \right] \quad (10.1)$$

From this expression it can be seen that as long as the ratio of the probability of a true positive to the probability of a false positive is sufficiently great, society will benefit from an approval regardless of the probability of a false positive. We can further rewrite this expression for the net benefit to society as

$$\sum_i p_0 \cdot \alpha \cdot \left[\frac{p_1}{p_0} \cdot \frac{\beta}{\alpha} \cdot A_i - B_i \right] \quad (10.2)$$

From this expression it can be deduced that the societal benefit from study i will be greater than zero if

$$\frac{\beta}{\alpha} > \frac{p_0 \cdot B_i}{p_1 \cdot A_i} \quad (10.3)$$

and the net societal benefit will be greater than zero if

$$\frac{\beta}{\alpha} > \frac{p_0 \cdot \sum_i B_i}{p_1 \cdot \sum_i A_i} = \frac{E(\text{Loss to Society})}{E(\text{Benefit to Society})} \quad (10.4)$$

Thus, an approval process will contribute to net societal benefit regardless of the absolute level of α if the ratio of power to type 1 error is sufficiently great.

It is interesting to note that the ratio of power to type 1 error is also a key quantity in determining the posterior probability that the drug is effective given a positive result, since by Bayes rule

$$p_{1,post} = \frac{p_{1,prior} \cdot \beta}{p_{1,prior} \cdot \beta + p_{0,prior} \cdot \alpha} \quad (10.5)$$

$$= \frac{p_{1,prior} \cdot \dfrac{\beta}{\alpha}}{p_{1,prior} \cdot \dfrac{\beta}{\alpha} + p_{0,prior}} \tag{10.6}$$

Further, one can also rephrase the Frequentist requirement that a trial have 80 percent power with a one-sided type 1 error of 0.025 as requiring that a trial have 80 percent power with a ratio of power to type 1 error of $0.80/0.025 = 32$.

10.1.2 Knowledge of p_0 and p_1

The calculation of the ratio of true to false positives requires knowledge of the probability of the null and alternative hypothesis. However, one does not need to know the probability of the null and alternative to be able to compare the ratio of true to false positives among two possible study designs or analyses in the same circumstances. That is, if we have two study designs or analyses with power β_1, β_2 and type 1 error α_1, α_2, then the ratio of true to false positives for the two situations will be related as

$$\frac{p_0 \cdot \beta_1}{p_1 \cdot \alpha_1} \propto \frac{p_0 \cdot \beta_2}{p_1 \cdot \alpha_2} \tag{10.7}$$

which will be true if and only if

$$\frac{\beta_1}{\alpha_1} \propto \frac{\beta_2}{\alpha_2} \tag{10.8}$$

In other words, the comparison of the ratio of true to false positives can be accomplished by simply comparing the ratio of power to type 1 error as long as it is reasonable to assume that p_0 and p_1 are the same.

10.1.3 Knowledge of the Treatment Effect Size

The calculation of the ratio of true to false positives also requires knowledge of the treatment effect size. In the development that follows, the magnitude of the treatment effect will be allowed to vary over a range of values. However, the key value for decision-making purposes is the minimum clinically meaningful difference (MCMD), the magnitude of the treatment effect that is typically used when calculating the sample size of a Phase 3 study. As long as the ratio of power to type 1 error is sufficiently great at the MCMD, the ratio of power to type 1 error will be sufficiently great for all treatment effect levels greater than the MCMD and hence for all θ in the alternative space corresponding to a treatment effect that is of benefit to patients. Essentially, this two-state model says that if the ratio of power to type 1 error is sufficiently great and the drug is approved, then the expected benefit arising from drugs that have a treatment effect size greater than or equal to the minimum clinically meaningful difference will be greater than the expected loss from drugs that have no treatment effect.

For treatment effect levels less than the MCMD consider the following three-state model that is a simple extension of the two-state model already introduced. In this model, if the drug is effective (T) the benefit to society is A, if the drug is not effective (F) the society loses B, and if the drug has activity that is greater than zero but less than the minimum clinically meaningful difference (o) the loss or benefit to society is 0. The existence of state (o) follows naturally from the assumption that the relationship between the treatment effect size and the net benefit to society from a drug approval is continuous. If this is the case, then there must be a treatment effect size between 0 and the MCMD, which results in a net societal benefit of 0.

Under this three-state model, the expected benefit to society from a drug approval is

$$P(+, T) \cdot A + P(+, o) \cdot 0 - P(+, F) \cdot B = P(+, F) \cdot \left[\frac{P(+, T)}{P(+, F)} \cdot A - B \right] \qquad (10.9)$$

In this three-state formulation of the decision problem the ratio of true to false positives is still key to determining whether the decision to reject the null hypothesis provides a net benefit to society. Thus, if we power a study so that the power divided by the type 1 error is sufficiently great at the MCMD, then we can deduce that even after accounting for true positive, false positive, and o positive approvals, society will benefit on average from an approval decision if the study is positive.

It is interesting to note that the hypothesis-testing framework is also based on quantifying the potential benefits and losses from decisions. In the first chapter of Lehmann (1959), he discusses the general decision problem as one of minimizing the expected loss. In hypothesis testing, the losses are set up by first dividing the parameter space into two subsets, H and A, each representing, respectively, the parameters in the probability model that are consistent with the null and alternative hypotheses. The loss function is defined to be 0 if the true state of nature and the decision based on data agree and 1 if they disagree. The expected loss is then the type 1 error if the state of nature is in H and it is the type 2 error if the state of nature is in A. The approach adopted in hypothesis testing to finding good decision functions is to set the type 1 error at an acceptable level and then attempt to minimize the type 2 error over all parameters in the alternative space A.

The notion of a minimum clinically meaningful difference cannot be incorporated into the loss functions for hypothesis testing as just described, since the losses are constant over the set A. Thus, we are left with a testing procedure that minimizes the type 2 error for all θ in A, even those θ that are less than the minimum clinically meaningful difference and that we are not interested in. So, the theoretical framework provided by hypothesis testing does not quite fit the decision problem we are faced with in clinical trials and hence we are left without a sound justification for decisions to approve or reject applications to market a new drug.

The three-stage model introduced in Equation (10.9) does directly incorporate the notion of a minimum clinically meaningful difference into the loss function and hence provides a theoretical foundation for the decisions regarding the marketing approval of new drugs. This is not to say that the mechanics of hypothesis testing are to be discarded. Rather that with the ideas introduced here we have a formal theoretical rationale for approving or rejecting drugs based on hypothesis tests.

10.2 Studies with Interim Analyses

Although describing the strength of a study's results with the ratio of power to type 1 error is very similar to the Bayesian and Frequentist approaches in the case of a study that is evaluated only once at the final analysis, differences start to emerge when one considers a trial with interim analyses. Indeed, the addition of interim analyses to a Phase 3 study adds complexity to the determination of the level of evidence that a positive study provides. For example, consider a simple O'Brien-Fleming boundary with three interim analyses and a final analysis. If the study stops at the first interim, the results are necessarily very strong in favor of the drug's activity because of the conservative nature of the O'Brien-Fleming stopping boundary at early interims. On the other hand, if the study is not positive until the final analysis, then the results will be much less favorable since the critical value for the final analysis of an O'Brien-Fleming stopping boundary is very close to the critical value for a study without any interims. Positive results, either at the first interim or the final analysis regardless of how discrepant they are, both lead to "statistical" rejection of the null hypothesis since the criteria for evaluating the evidence from such a study involves the type 1 error for the study as a whole. As long as the probability of exceeding the rejection boundary for the study as a whole under the null hypothesis is 0.025 and under the alternative is 0.80, the evidence from the study is considered positive. Such a criteria for determining whether the study is positive does not quantify the level of evidence supporting marketing approval at each individual analysis.

10.2.1 Ratio of True to False Positives Given Where the Study Stopped

To illustrate how the strength of evidence provided by a study that stops at an interim analysis is quantified by the ratio of power to type 1 error, let's consider a study with a single interim analysis. Table 10.1 describes the notation

TABLE 10.1

Probability of Rejecting the Null Hypothesis: Notation

	Prior Probability	Interim	Final	Overall
H_0	$1-p$	α_1	α_2	$\alpha_1 + \alpha_2$
H_A	p	β_1	β_2	$\beta_1 + \beta_2$

for the power and type 1 error at each analysis point. The column labeled "Interim" presents the probability of exceeding the rejection boundary at the first analysis. The column labeled "Final" presents the probability of not crossing the rejection boundary at the first analysis and subsequently crossing the rejection boundary at the final analysis. Last, the column labeled "Overall" presents the probability of crossing the boundary for the study as a whole, that is, either at the interim or the final analysis.

The expected benefit to society of a rejection at any time is

$$p \cdot (\beta_1 + \beta_2) \cdot A - (1-p) \cdot (\alpha_1 + \alpha_2) \cdot B$$

$$= (\alpha_1 + \alpha_2) \cdot \left[p \cdot \frac{\beta_1 + \beta_2}{\alpha_1 + \alpha_2} \cdot A - (1-p) \cdot B \right] \qquad (10.10)$$

This benefit will be positive if

$$\frac{\beta_1 + \beta_2}{\alpha_1 + \alpha_2} > \frac{B}{A} \cdot \frac{1-p}{p} \qquad (10.11)$$

that is, if the total power divided by the total type 1 error is sufficiently great. The practice of designing a study with overall power of 80 percent and overall type 1 error of 0.025 will provide a net benefit to society when averaged over repeated outcomes of the study if the ratio of power to type 1 error, in this case $0.80/0.025 = 32$, is great enough. Unfortunately, although the average benefit across all possible outcomes for the study may be positive it is possible that the benefit averaged only over outcomes where the study rejects at the first analysis is positive and the benefit averaged only over outcomes where the study rejects at the last analysis is negative or vice versa. To further define this possibility we will calculate the expected benefit to society of a rejection at each analysis in the example described by Table 10.1.

The expected benefit to society given that the study stopped at the interim is calculated by first determining the probability that the drug is or is not effective conditional on this stopping point:

$$P(+, T / \text{Stop at Interim 1}) = \frac{p \cdot \beta_1}{p \cdot \beta_1 + (1-p) \cdot \alpha_1} \qquad (10.12)$$

$$P(+, F/\text{Stop at Interim 1}) = \frac{(1-p)\cdot\alpha_1}{p\cdot\beta_1 + (1-p)\cdot\alpha_1} \tag{10.13}$$

The expected benefit to society from a study that stopped at the interim is thus

$$\frac{p\cdot\beta_1}{p\cdot\beta_1 + (1-p)\cdot\alpha_1}\cdot A - \frac{(1-p)\cdot\alpha_1}{p\cdot\beta_1 + (1-p)\cdot\alpha_1}\cdot B \tag{10.14}$$

$$= \frac{(1-p)\cdot\alpha_1}{p\cdot\beta_1 + (1-p)\cdot\alpha_1}\cdot\left[\frac{p\cdot\beta_1}{(1-p)\cdot\alpha_1}\cdot A - B\right] \tag{10.15}$$

The expected benefit conditional on the study stopping at the interim will be positive provided that

$$\frac{p\cdot\beta_1}{(1-p)\cdot\alpha_1}\cdot A - B > 0 \qquad \text{or} \qquad \frac{\beta_1}{\alpha_1} > \frac{B}{A}\cdot\frac{1-p}{p} \tag{10.16}$$

Similarly, the expected benefit given the study stopped at the final analysis is positive if

$$\frac{p\cdot\beta_2}{(1-p)\cdot\alpha_2}\cdot A - B > 0 \qquad \text{or} \qquad \frac{\beta_2}{\alpha_2} > \frac{B}{A}\cdot\frac{1-p}{p} \tag{10.17}$$

So society will benefit from those drugs that are approved based on studies that stopped and rejected the null hypothesis at the interim analysis if the ratio of power to type 1 error at the interim is sufficiently great. What's more, the level that the ratio of power to type 1 error must exceed in order to provide a net benefit to society is the same at each analysis and for the study as a whole. Further, if the ratio of power to type 1 error for the study as a whole equals 32 and this ratio is not constant at each analysis, then necessarily the ratio of power to type 1 error will be greater than 32 for some analyses and less than 32 for others. That is, although society will benefit on average from a positive study regardless of where it crosses the rejection boundary, there will be some interims where the expected benefit to society from a positive result is negative.

10.2.2 A Constant Ratio of Cumulative Power to Cumulative Type 1 Error Is Equivalent to a Constant Ratio of True to False Positives Given Where the Study Stopped

As discussed earlier, if the study is calibrated so that the ratio of overall power to overall type 1 error is sufficient to ensure that society will benefit on average from an approval decision, then the condition that the ratio of power to type 1 error given where the study stops equals a constant at every analysis ensures that the net benefit to society of a positive study and subsequent approval decision is positive regardless of where the study stops. However, this ratio of power to type 1 error given where the study stops is not monotone increasing as a function of the treatment effect size, which makes it difficult to form a rule for declaring that the study is positive. Fortunately, the ratio of the cumulative power to the cumulative type 1 error is monotone increasing. What's more, the property that the ratio of power to type 1 error conditional on where the study stopped is constant at each analysis is equivalent to the ratio of the cumulative power to the cumulative type 1 error being constant at each analysis. Additionally, it can be further stated that a constant ratio of cumulative power to cumulative type 1 error at each analysis is equivalent to the ratio of true positives to false positives conditional on where the study stopped being a constant at all analyses. We show this formally next.

Let α_j and β_j denote the cumulative type 1 error and the cumulative power at the jth analysis. Assume that $\beta_j = C \cdot \alpha_j$ for all j. Then

$$P(+, T/\text{Stop at } I_j) = \frac{P(+, \text{Stop at } I_j / T) \cdot P(T)}{P(\text{Stop at } I_j / T) \cdot P(T) + P(\text{Stop at } I_j / F) \cdot P(F)} \tag{10.18}$$

and similarly

$$P(+, F/\text{Stop at } I_j) = \frac{P(+, \text{Stop at } I_j / F) \cdot P(F)}{P(\text{Stop at } I_j / T) \cdot P(T) + P(\text{Stop at } I_j / F) \cdot P(F)} \tag{10.19}$$

So

$$\frac{P(+, T/\text{Stop at } I_j)}{P(+, F/\text{Stop at } I_j)} = \frac{P(+, \text{Stop at } I_j / T) \cdot P(T)}{P(+, \text{Stop at } I_j / F) \cdot P(F)} = \frac{\beta_j - \beta_{j-1}}{\alpha_j - \alpha_{j-1}} \cdot \frac{p_1}{p_0} \tag{10.20}$$

$$= \frac{C \cdot \alpha_j - C \cdot \alpha_{j-1}}{\alpha_j - \alpha_{j-1}} \cdot \frac{p_1}{p_0} = C \cdot \frac{p_1}{p_0} \tag{10.21}$$

So, if the ratio of cumulative power to cumulative type 1 error is the same at each analysis, then the ratio of true positives to false positives conditional on where the study stopped is the same at each analysis as well.

Suppose conversely that the ratio of true positives to false positives conditional on where the study stopped is equal to a constant C at each analysis. That is

$$\frac{P(+, T/\text{Stop at } I_j)}{P(+, F/\text{Stop at } I_j)} = C \tag{10.22}$$

Then

$$C = \frac{P(+, \text{Stop at } I_j/T) \cdot P(T)}{P(+, \text{Stop at } I_j/F) \cdot P(F)} = \frac{\beta_j - \beta_{j-1}}{\alpha_j - \alpha_{j-1}} \cdot \frac{p_1}{p_0} \tag{10.23}$$

We will proceed by induction. First, note that from Equation (10.23) with $j = 1$, we have

$$\beta_1 = \frac{p_0}{p_1} C \cdot \alpha_1 \tag{10.24}$$

Now if $\beta_i = \frac{p_0}{p_1} C \alpha_i$, then since

$$\frac{\beta_{i+1} - \beta_i}{\alpha_{i+1} - \alpha_i} \cdot \frac{p_1}{p_0} = C \tag{10.25}$$

we can infer

$$\beta_{i+1} - \beta_i = \frac{p_0}{p_1} \cdot C \cdot (\alpha_{i+1} - \alpha_i) \tag{10.26}$$

$$\beta_{i+1} - \frac{p_0}{p_1} \cdot C \cdot \alpha_i = \frac{p_0}{p_1} \cdot C \cdot (\alpha_{i+1} - \alpha_i) \tag{10.27}$$

$$\beta_{i+1} = \frac{p_0}{p_1} \cdot C \cdot \alpha_{i+1} \tag{10.28}$$

So, by induction we have that

$$\beta_i = \frac{p_0}{p_1} C \alpha_i \qquad \text{for all } i \tag{10.29}$$

or

$$\frac{\beta_i}{\alpha_i} = \frac{p_0}{p_1} \cdot C \qquad \text{for all } i \tag{10.30}$$

Thus, the requirement that the ratio of true positives to false positives conditional on where the study stops is the same at each analysis is equivalent to requiring that the rejection boundary be such that the cumulative power divided by the cumulative type 1 error is the same at each analysis.

It is interesting to note that Wald's (1947) sequential probability ratio test has the property that the ratio of power to type 1 error at each analysis exceeds a specified level. This mirrors the requirements that we developed here from considering the ratio of true to false positives.

Designing interim analyses based on the ratio of power to type 1 error does not preclude this ratio from being unequal at the various analysis times.

One can directly specify the ratio of power to type 1 error conditional on stopping at an interim analysis to be whatever seems appropriate and as long as these ratios at the minimum clinically meaningful difference are greater than 32 the boundary would be acceptable. That is, the boundary would result in decisions that lead to a net societal benefit regardless of where the study stopped.

10.3 A Boundary with a Constant Ratio of Power to Type 1 Error

Table 10.2 and Figure 10.1 present an example of a rejection boundary constructed to maintain the ratio of power to type 1 error at a fixed level, 32, at each of seven analyses in conjunction with a Pocock futility boundary. The power was evaluated at the targeted treatment effect size of 0.315. Thirty-two was chosen for the ratio of power to type 1 error since it represents the ratio of power to type 1 error in a typically powered Phase 3 study, that is, 0.80/0.025. Table 10.2 provides basic information regarding the power and type 1 error at each analysis, and Figure 10.1 presents as a function of the treatment effect size, the cumulative power, the ratio of the cumulative power to the cumulative type 1 error, and the ratio of the change in power to the change in the

TABLE 10.2

An Example of an Interim Analysis Boundary with a Constant Ratio of Power to Type 1 Error

	Interim 1	Interim 2	Interim 3	Interim 4	Interim 5	Interim 6	Final Analysis
Number of subjects per group	21	43	64	86	107	129	150
Z-statistic (reject the null)	2.73	2.28	2.28	2.34	2.42	2.51	2.59
Z-statistic (reject the alt)	−1.03	−0.43	0.04	0.43	0.77	1.08	1.37
Cumulative power	0.102	0.425	0.632	0.762	0.843	0.893	0.924
Cumulative type 1 error (one-sided)	0.0032	0.0133	0.0198	0.0238	0.0263	0.0279	0.0289
β/α	32	31.99	31.99	32	32	32	32
$\Delta\beta/\Delta\alpha$	—	31.99	31.99	32.04	31.97	32.02	32.02
Effect size	0.315						

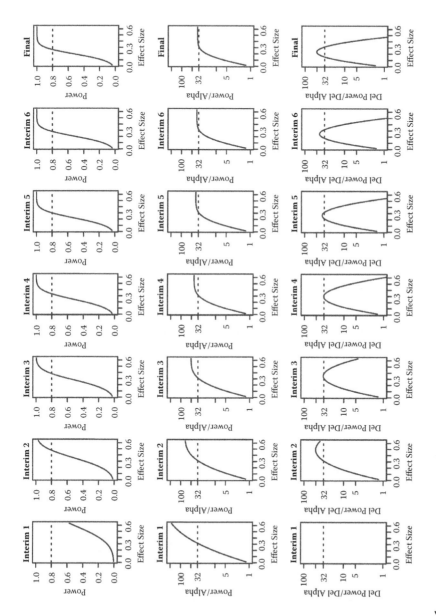

FIGURE 10.1
Operating characteristics of the stopping boundary in Table 10.2.

type 1 error in moving from one analysis to the next, ΔPower/ΔType 1 error, or equivalently $\dfrac{\beta_j - \beta_{j-1}}{\alpha_j - \alpha_{j-1}}$. Recall that ΔPower/ΔType 1 at the ith interim is the same as the ratio of power to type 1 error conditional on the study stopping at the ith interim analysis.

10.3.1 Properties

As described in Table 10.2, type 1 error of 0.025 is exceeded at the fifth analysis, whereas the type 1 error of the study at the last analysis is 0.029 with power of 0.924. Further, the rejection boundary represented by the Z-statistic is larger at the first analysis than at all other analyses. The evidential requirement in terms of the Z-test is relaxed at the second analysis but increases thereafter with the number of analyses.

It can be seen in Figure 10.1 that the ratio of power to type 1 error is monotone increasing as a function of the treatment effect size. The situation is different for ΔPower/ΔType 1 error. This ratio is not monotonically increasing as a function of the treatment effect size, θ, for interim analyses following the first one. For analyses two and three the interval where the ratio of power to type 1 error is greater than 32 has the targeted treatment effect size as its left endpoint. For analyses four, five, six, and seven this interval has the targeted treatment effect size as its right-hand endpoint.

10.3.2 ΔPower/ΔType 1 Error as an Unbiased Test

An unbiased test is one whose power, β, is greater than the level of the test, α, for all θ in the alternative. In terms of the ratio of power to type 1 error, an unbiased test must have Power/Type 1 error > 1 for θ in the alternative. The observation that ΔPower/ΔType 1 error is not monotonically increasing and in fact is decreasing to zero as $\theta \to \infty$ means we cannot interpret a test based on ΔPower/ΔType 1 error as an unbiased test of H_0: $\theta = 0$ versus H_A: $\theta > 0$. However, a test at analysis j based on ΔPower/ΔType 1 error can be viewed as an unbiased test of $(\theta \le \theta_0) \cup (\theta \in A_j^+)$ versus $(\theta > \theta_0) \cap (\theta \in A_j^+)^c$ where $A_j^+ = \left\{ \theta > \theta_0 : \dfrac{\beta_j(\theta) - \beta_{j-1}(\theta)}{\alpha_j - \alpha_{j-1}} \le 1 \right\}$. Thus, crossing the rejection boundary at analysis j would lead one to conclude that θ is not a null treatment effect and θ is not a treatment effect larger than the left-hand endpoint of A_j^+, but rather θ is a treatment effect in $(\theta > \theta_0) \cap A_j^{+c}$.

Since the boundary in this example was constructed so that the ratio β_j/α_j at the targeted treatment effect size is 32 at each interim analysis, the set B_j defined by

$$B_j = \left\{ \theta : \dfrac{\beta_j(\theta) - \beta_{j-1}(\theta)}{\alpha_j - \alpha_{j-1}} \ge 32 \right\} \tag{10.31}$$

is not empty. Here, I_j denotes the event of the study stopping at interim j. Thus, there are $\theta \in B_j$ where the ratio of ΔPower to ΔType 1 error is greater than 32.

However, when $\min_{\theta \in B_j} \theta$ no longer represents a treatment effect of clinical benefit, then a "positive" study result at interim j no longer allows one to distinguish a meaningful benefit from a meaningless one. The desire to avoid this situation would lead to an indirect limit on the sample size of such a study. This example shows that it is important to monitor the ratio ΔPower/ΔType 1 error to be sure that the power that is being added at each interim is associated with meaningful evidence that the drug is effective. The next example, an O'Brien-Fleming stopping boundary, makes the same point in a different way.

10.4 O'Brien-Fleming Boundary

Table 10.3 provides the ratios of the cumulative power to cumulative type 1 error for an O'Brien-Fleming stopping boundary along with changes in these quantities in moving from one analysis to the next. Figure 10.2 provides graphs of these quantities over a range of treatment effect sizes.

10.4.1 Lack of Evidence at the Final Analysis

As seen in Table 10.3, the ratio of power at the targeted treatment effect size to type 1 error for this O'Brien-Fleming boundary is much greater at the early interims than it is at the final analysis. Further, the ratio of power to type 1 error is slightly greater than 32 at the final analysis. However, at the final analysis, the ratio of power to type 1 error at the targeted treatment effect size conditional on stopping at the final analysis is less than half of 32. What's more, as shown in Figure 10.2, the maximum of the ratio of power to type 1 error over all θ conditional on stopping at the final analysis is also less than half of 32 at the final analysis. Thus, at the last analysis of this O'Brien-Fleming boundary, the set

$$B_{Final} = \left\{ \theta : \frac{\beta_{Final}(\theta) - \beta_{Final-1}(\theta)}{\alpha_{Final} - \alpha_{Final-1}} \geq 32 \right\} \qquad (10.32)$$

is empty, meaning that the test conditional on stopping at the last analysis of this stopping boundary could not support the rejection of the null hypothesis with a ratio of power to type 1 error greater than 32 for any θ. So, while stopping at the early interims provides very strong evidence in favor of a drug's activity, stopping at the last analysis provides very weak evidence of activity, much weaker than is provided by a similar study with no interims. We can evaluate this formally as follows.

TABLE 10.3

An Example of an O'Brien-Fleming Stopping Boundary

	Interim 1	Interim 2	Interim 3	Interim 4	Final Analysis
Number of subjects per group	16	33	49	65	82
Z-statistic	4.57	3.23	2.64	2.28	2.04
Cumulative power	0	0.077	0.337	0.614	0.802
Cumulative type 1 error (one-sided)	0	0.001	0.004	0.013	0.025
β/α	—	77	84.25	47.23	32.08
$\Delta\beta/\Delta\alpha$	—	77	86.67	30.78	15.67
Effect size	0.315				

The distribution of positives between those that are true and those that are false given the study stopped at an interim is described by the following two equations

$$P(T,+/I) = \frac{\beta_N(\theta) \cdot f(\theta)}{\alpha_N \cdot f(\theta_0) + \int \beta_N(\theta) \cdot f(\theta) \cdot d\theta} \tag{10.33}$$

$$P(F,+/I) = \frac{\alpha_N \cdot f(\theta_0)}{\alpha_N \cdot f(\theta_0) + \int \beta_N(\theta) \cdot f(\theta) \cdot d\theta} \tag{10.34}$$

The expected benefit of the decision rule if the study stops at interim I is thus

$$E(Benefit / I) = A \cdot \frac{\int \beta_N(\theta) \cdot f(\theta) \cdot d\theta}{\alpha_N \cdot f(\theta_0) + \int \beta_N(\theta) \cdot f(\theta) \cdot d\theta} -$$

$$B \cdot \frac{\alpha_N \cdot f(\theta_0)}{\alpha_N \cdot f(\theta_0) + \int \beta_N(\theta) \cdot f(\theta) \cdot d\theta} \tag{10.35}$$

$$= \frac{\alpha_N \cdot f(\theta_0)}{\alpha_N \cdot f(\theta_0) + \int \beta_N(\theta) \cdot f(\theta) \cdot d\theta} \cdot \left\{ A \cdot \int \frac{\beta_N(\theta)}{\alpha_N \cdot f(\theta_0)} \cdot f(\theta) \cdot d\theta - B \right\} \tag{10.36}$$

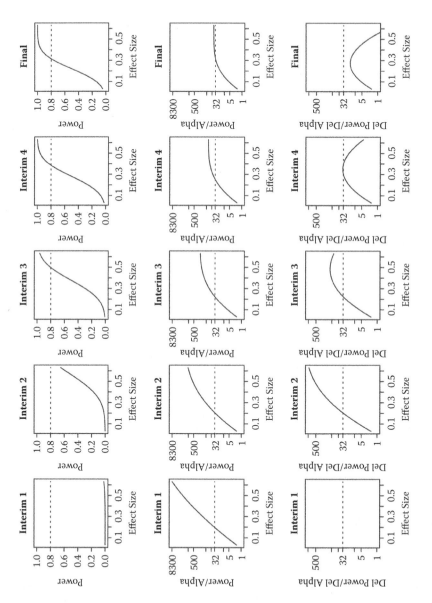

FIGURE 10.2
Operating characteristics of an O'Brien-Fleming stopping boundary.

while the expected benefit without conditioning on the interim is

$$
E(Benefit) = A \cdot \frac{\int \beta(\theta) \cdot f(\theta) \cdot d\theta}{\alpha \cdot f(\theta_0) + \int \beta(\theta) \cdot f(\theta) \cdot d\theta} - B \cdot \frac{\alpha \cdot f(\theta_0)}{\alpha \cdot f(\theta_0) + \int \beta(\theta) \cdot f(\theta) \cdot d\theta}
$$

(10.37)

$$
= \frac{\alpha \cdot f(\theta_0)}{\alpha \cdot f(\theta_0) + \int \beta(\theta) \cdot f(\theta) \cdot d\theta} \cdot \left\{ A \cdot \int \frac{\beta(\theta)}{\alpha \cdot f(\theta_0)} \cdot f(\theta) \cdot d\theta - B \right\} \quad (10.38)
$$

So if $\dfrac{\beta(\theta)}{\alpha}$ for the study as a whole is at the minimum level necessary to ensure that

$$
A \cdot \int \frac{\beta(\theta)}{\alpha} \cdot \frac{f(\theta)}{f(\theta_0)} \cdot d\theta - B > 0
$$

(10.39)

then $\dfrac{\beta_N(\theta)}{\alpha_N}$ which is less than half what it is for the study as a whole for $\theta \geq$, the minimum clinically meaningful difference, is not at a level that will guarantee a positive expected benefit for society from an approval decision.

To see what the low ratio of power to type 1 error at the final analysis means in practice, suppose that we have a Phase 3 study of an oncology drug with such an interim analysis plan that stops at the final analysis with significant results. In Chapter 12, we estimate the probability that a Phase 3 study of an oncology drug will be successful is 53 percent. Using this estimate, the ratio of true positives to false positives conditional on stopping at the last analysis would be less than $0.53 \times 16 = 8.48$, or the proportion of these studies that are false positives would be more than $1/(1 + 8.48) = 0.105$.

10.4.2 Evidence at Early Analyses

Now let's look at the results for interims 1, 2, and 3. For all of these interims the ratio of power to type 1 error conditional on the study stopping at that point is much greater than 32 over a wide range of θ that includes the targeted treatment effect size. As we move from the first to the third interim analysis, the ratio of power to type 1 error conditional on where the study stopped decreases and by the fourth analysis is less than 32. It is precisely the high ratio of power to type 1 error at these early interims that leads to the lack of evidence in favor of the drug if the O'Brien-Fleming boundary is crossed at the final analysis.

10.4.3 Discussion

Proponents of the O'Brien-Fleming boundary might say that a study that made it to the end and crossed the rejection boundary at the last analysis would also have been positive had there not been a plan for interim analyses. That is, practically speaking, the same sample paths that would lead to rejection at the final analysis with an O'Brien-Fleming boundary would also lead to rejection in the same study without an interim analysis plan. In this sense, the level of evidence that is required for an approval does not change whether or not there is an interim analysis employed in the trial. However, interim analyses in a study provide information about the treatment effect of the drug and our certainty about the effectiveness of drugs that are only positive at the last analysis may not be as good as is desired if the final analysis follows a series of interims that require large treatment effects to stop the study, as with an O'Brien-Fleming boundary.

More generally, proponents of the Frequentist paradigm underlying the use of interim analysis in clinical trials might say that the cumulative type 1 error at any interim analysis will always be less than 0.025 as in a study with only one analysis and that the cumulative power will be at least 0.80 for some alternative. So, if a study stops at an interim analysis, the evidence in favor of drug approval will always be consistent with the evidence provided by a study with a single analysis. But to support regulatory approval the power has to be sufficient at the minimal clinically meaningful difference as well. Otherwise the regulator and society will be assuming additional risk that the drug is not effective beyond what they are prepared to accept, which may lead to a net reduction in expected societal benefit. And as noted before, it is the responsibility of the sponsor to reduce the risk to a level that is acceptable to the regulator.

Alternatively, Frequentist proponents may say that as long as the overall type 1 error is 0.025 and the overall power for the study at the minimum clinically meaningful difference is at least 80 percent, the study should be considered positive regardless of which analysis the study stopped at. With this view, the level of evidence that will lead to the study stopping at the first interim analysis depends on the level of evidence at which the study will be stopped for all the interim analyses that follow. One cannot look simply at the data collected and the associated rules for stopping the study at that point and say what the strength of evidence is. One has to look also at the plan for evaluating data at all of the following interim analyses to judge how strong the evidence is, which is very nonintuitive. Such an approach does not provide a reasonable assessment of the strength of evidence at each interim.

In summary, allowing any sort of stopping boundaries to be constructed as long as the power for the trial as a whole is 80 percent and the type 1 error for the study as a whole is 0.025 means that the level of evidence may be higher at some analyses and lower at others. And the level of evidence may be even lower than would be expected for a study conducted without any interim analyses.

10.5 Bayesian or Frequentist?

Now we compare the evaluation of the evidence from a clinical trial based on the ratio of true to false positives with the two main statistical approaches to the evaluation of data, namely, Bayesian and Frequentist.

10.5.1 Formal Comparison with the Bayesian Approach

If we let $f(\theta)$ be a prior on the size of the treatment effect, θ, the ratio of true to false positives can be written in general as

$$\frac{\int_{\theta \in T} P(+ \text{ and Stop at } I_i \mid \theta) \cdot f(\theta) \cdot d\theta}{\int_{\theta \in F} P(+ \text{ and Stop at } I_i \mid \theta) \cdot f(\theta) \cdot d\theta} \tag{10.40}$$

This quantity is related to the posterior probability that $\theta \in T$, which is the value commonly used in the Bayesian framework to determine if a drug is effective. To see this note that if $\{\theta \in T\} \cup \{\theta \in F\} = R$ and the Bayesian posterior distribution is written as

$$\frac{f(x \mid \theta) \cdot f(\theta)}{\int_{-\infty}^{\infty} f(x \mid \theta) \cdot f(\theta) \cdot d\theta} \tag{10.41}$$

then

$$h[P(\theta \in T \mid x)] = \frac{P(\theta \in T \mid x)}{P(\theta \in F \mid x)}$$

$$= \frac{\int_{\theta \in T} \dfrac{f(x \mid \theta) \cdot f(\theta)}{\int_{-\infty}^{\infty} f(x \mid \theta) \cdot f(\theta) \cdot d\theta} \cdot d\theta}{\int_{\theta \in F} \dfrac{f(x \mid \theta) \cdot f(\theta)}{\int_{-\infty}^{\infty} f(x \mid \theta) \cdot f(\theta) \cdot d\theta} \cdot d\theta} = \frac{\int_{\theta \in T} f(x \mid \theta) \cdot f(\theta) \cdot d\theta}{\int_{\theta \in F} f(x \mid \theta) \cdot f(\theta) \cdot d\theta} \tag{10.42}$$

where $h(x) = x/(1 - x)$. Since h is a monotone increasing function, the Bayesian criteria of stopping if the posterior probability that $\theta \in T$ is greater than some quantity is equivalent to requiring that the ratio of the posterior probability the drug is effective to the posterior probability the drug is not effective exceeds some threshold. And as shown in Equation (10.42), the ratio of the posterior probabilities reduces to the ratio of the probabilities that the data x is observed under the null and alternative. Thus, the difference between evaluating a drug based on the ratio of true to false positives and based on the Bayesian framework is simply that $P(+ \text{ and Stop at } I_i|\theta)$ is substituted for $f(x/\theta)$ in the Bayesian framework. The use of $P(+ \text{ and Stop at } I_i|\theta)$ instead of $f(x/\theta)$ is motivated by Frequentist considerations.

10.5.2 Are These Approaches to Evaluating the Strength of Evidence Different? An Example

Although the formulaic difference with a Bayesian analysis seems minor, the following example illustrates that the two approaches can lead to different conclusions. Consider a study designed with two analyses as described in Table 10.4 and Table 10.5. The impact of the futility boundary on the power and type 1 error can be seen in the tables and is sometimes described as "buying back alpha." As described in Table 10.4, the stopping boundary without the futility boundary would result in type 1 error for the study as a whole of 0.025. However, adding a futility boundary that requires a positive trend early "buys back" alpha resulting in the actual type 1 error for the study being 0.014, as reported in Table 10.5.

Now let's consider how a Bayesian would evaluate data from this study. First, assume that the Bayesian prior distribution on the size of the treatment effect is a normal distribution with mean zero and variance such that the probability the treatment effect is greater than the minimum clinically meaningful difference, 0.20, is 0.10. That is, the prior on the treatment effect, $(\mu_T - \mu_C)/\sqrt{2 \cdot \sigma^2}$, is a normal distribution with mean zero and variance 0.02437. Let's further assume that the Bayesian criteria based on the posterior distribution for the treatment effect is calibrated so that it would declare the drug is effective if a simple 80 percent powered trial with a single analysis and a one-sided type 1 error of 0.025 is positive. Now a study with 80 percent power at a one-sided type 1 error of 0.025 and a treatment

TABLE 10.4

Example: No Futility Boundary

	Interim 1	Final Analysis
Number of subjects per group	65	131
Z-statistic (reject the null)	6	1.959
Z-statistic (reject the alt)	−5	1.959
Cumulative power	0	0.6293
Cumulative type 1 error (one-sided)	0	0.0251
β/α	5809.69	25.12
$\Delta\beta/\Delta\alpha$	0	25.12
Effect size	0.2	

TABLE 10.5

Example: Futility Boundary

	Interim 1	Final Analysis
Number of subjects per group	65	131
Z-statistic (reject the null)	6	1.959
Z-statistic (reject the alt)	1.51	1.959
Cumulative power	0	0.4577
Cumulative type 1 error (one-sided)	0	0.0143
Cumulative probability of stopping for futility (alt)	0.4592	0.5423
Cumulative probability of stopping for futility (null)	0.9345	0.9857
β/α	5809.69	32.09
$\Delta\beta/\Delta\alpha$	0	32.09
Effect size	0.2	

effect size of 0.20 requires 196 subjects. So, the posterior distribution on the treatment effect after observing a Z-statistic of 1.96 associated with such a study has mean

$$\frac{\dfrac{1.96/\sqrt{196}}{1/196}+\dfrac{0.00}{0.02437}}{\dfrac{1}{1/196}+\dfrac{1}{0.02437}}=0.1158 \tag{10.43}$$

and variance

$$\frac{1}{\dfrac{1}{1/196}+\dfrac{1}{0.02437}}=0.004219 \tag{10.44}$$

and the posterior probability that the treatment effect is less than zero is then

$$\Phi\left(\frac{0-0.1158}{\sqrt{0.004219}}\right)=0.03731 \tag{10.45}$$

So, a Bayesian who is consistent with a Frequentist evaluation of the final analysis of an 80 percent powered trial with type 1 error of 0.025 would declare the drug effective if the posterior probability that the treatment is the same or inferior to control (effect size is less than zero) is less than 0.037.

The posterior mean and variance were calculated based on the following formula. Let the prior be normally distributed with mean, μ_{prior} and variance σ^2_{prior}. And let the data, X, be normally distributed with mean μ_{data} and variance σ^2_{data}. Then if we observe X, the posterior is normally distributed with mean and variance

$$\mu_{post} = \frac{X/\sigma^2_{data} + \mu_{prior}/\sigma^2_{prior}}{1/\sigma^2_{data} + 1/\sigma^2_{prior}} \tag{10.46}$$

$$\sigma^2_{post} = \frac{1}{1/\sigma^2_{data} + 1/\sigma^2_{prior}} \tag{10.47}$$

Now let's suppose that the data generated by the trial described by either Table 10.4 or Table 10.5 was a Z-statistic of 1.6 at the first analysis and 1.98 at the final analysis. Then the posterior distribution at the interim will have mean

$$\frac{\dfrac{1.6/\sqrt{65}}{1/65} + \dfrac{0}{0.02437}}{\dfrac{1}{1/65} + \dfrac{1}{0.02437}} = 0.1217 \tag{10.48}$$

and variance

$$\frac{1}{\dfrac{1}{1/65} + \dfrac{1}{0.02437}} = 0.009431 \tag{10.49}$$

and the posterior probability that the treatment effect size is less than zero is

$$\Phi\left(\frac{0 - 0.1217}{\sqrt{0.009431}}\right) = 0.1052 \tag{10.50}$$

Similarly, at the final analysis the posterior mean and variance will be, respectively,

$$\frac{\dfrac{1.200/\sqrt{65}}{1/65} + \dfrac{0.1217}{0.009431}}{\dfrac{1}{1/65} + \dfrac{1}{0.009431}} = 0.1320 \tag{10.51}$$

and

$$\frac{1}{\dfrac{1}{1/65} + \dfrac{1}{0.009431}} = 0.005847 \tag{10.52}$$

and the posterior probability that the treatment effect size is less than zero is

$$\Phi\left(\frac{0-0.1320}{\sqrt{0.005847}}\right) = 0.04215 \tag{10.53}$$

Thus, at both the interim and the final analysis the Bayesian would not support marketing approval because the posterior probability that the treatment effect size is less than zero is greater than 0.0374. Note that the Z-statistic of 1.200 that we used in Equation (10.51) to calculate the posterior distribution at the final analysis is meant to summarize only the data collected following the interim analysis. As such, it is consistent with a Z of 1.98 at the final analysis and a Z of 1.6 at the interim since

$$\frac{1.65 \cdot \sqrt{65} + 1.200 \cdot \sqrt{65}}{\sqrt{130}} = 1.98 \tag{10.54}$$

An analysis based on the ratio of power to type 1 error indicates as well that this data without the futility boundary would not support marketing approval. However, if the data were collected in the context of a study with a futility boundary of 1.51 at the first analysis, the results would support marketing approval with a ratio of power to type 1 error of 32 at the final analysis. The difference with the Bayesian approach is due to the fact that the Bayesian analysis ignores the rejection and futility boundaries (Berry 1985), whereas the analysis based on the ratio of power to type 1 error does not. That is, the futility boundary reduces the power of the study and reduces the type 1 error proportionally even more. This increases the likelihood that the observed results are due to an active treatment and the Bayesian analysis does not account for this. It should be noted that a Frequentist would also consider the result of this study not significant with or without the futility boundary since the overall power is less than 80 percent. This difference with the Frequentist approach arises because the Frequentist focuses on the power for the study as a whole rather than the evidence at each individual analysis.

This example demonstrates that the "statistical" evaluation of the results of a study, whether Bayesian or Frequentist, may not provide a complete assessment of the evidence in favor or against granting marketing approval to a new drug. Indeed, incorporating power into the Frequentist assessment of the results of a clinical trial as we have proposed here adds to the understanding of the evidence generated by a clinical trial beyond the typical statistical evaluations of the results of a study.

What's more, this example serves as a nice prelude to Chapter 12, which looks at the strength of evidence across Phase 2 and Phase 3 in total. A study design with a single futility analysis preceding the final analysis as in this example can be thought of as a Phase 2 trial that precedes a Phase 3 trial. The analysis of the Phase 2 trial results corresponds to the futility analysis, while the pooled analysis of Phase 2 and Phase 3 combined corresponds to the final analysis of the study. The ability of the ratio of power to type 1 error to capture the impact of a futility boundary also allows it to quantify the strength of evidence provided by a Phase 2/Phase 3 clinical program. This is a feature of the ratio of true to false positives that is not shared by the Bayesian or Frequentist approaches to evaluating evidence.

Finally, Appendix C proves an important property of the ratio of true to false positives, namely, that if the rejection boundary for the study is set such that the result of the study, X, lies on the boundary, then $\beta(X)/\alpha(X)$ increases monotonically to $+\infty$ as X goes to $+\infty$. This is a property that a measure of the strength of evidence should have.

References

Berry, D.A. 1985. Interim analysis in clinical trials: Classical vs. Bayesian approaches. *Stat Med* 4:521–526.

Lehmann, E.L. 1959. *Testing Statistical Hypotheses*. New York: Wiley.

O'Brien, P.C., Fleming, T.R. 1979. A multiple testing procedure for clinical trials. *Biometrics* 35:549–556.

Pocock, S.J. 1977. Group sequential methods in the design and analysis of clinical trials. *Biometrika* 64(2):191–199.

Wald, A. 1947. *Sequential Analysis*. New York: Dover.

11

Quantifying the Strength of Evidence: A Few Additional Comments on Interim Analyses

This chapter discusses a few more aspects of interim analyses, in particular Wald's likelihood ratio test and Pocock's stopping boundary for group sequential clinical trials.

11.1 Wald's Likelihood Ratio Test

As we noted in Chapter 10, Wald's likelihood ratio test has the property that the ratio of the power at a specific alternative to the type 1 error is greater than or equal to a constant. To see this, note that Wald's likelihood ratio test can be described as follows. Let X be distributed as $f_\theta(x)$. Then to distinguish between the null hypothesis θ_0 and the alternative θ_1 we form the likelihood ratio at each evaluation j and compare it to a constant r.

$$\frac{\prod\limits_{i=1}^{Nj} f_{\theta_1}(x)}{\prod\limits_{i=1}^{Nj} f_{\theta_0}(x)} > r \tag{11.1}$$

If the likelihood ratio is greater than r, then we reject the null hypothesis. Now the incremental probability of rejecting the null hypothesis under the alternative at each analysis is

$$\int\limits_{\text{Rejection Region}_j} \left[\prod\limits_{i=1}^{Nj} f_{\theta_1}(x_i) \right] \cdot dx_1 \ldots dx_{N_j} > \int\limits_{\text{Rejection Region}_j} \left[r \cdot \prod\limits_{i=1}^{Nj} f_{\theta_0}(x_i) \right] \cdot dx_1 \ldots dx_{N_j} \tag{11.2}$$

$$= r \cdot \int\limits_{\text{RejectionRegion}_j} \left[\prod\limits_{i=1}^{Nj} f_{\theta_0}(x_i) \right] \cdot dx_1 \ldots dx_{N_j} \tag{11.3}$$

and so

$$\frac{\text{Power}_j}{\text{Type 1 error}_j} = \frac{\displaystyle\int_{\text{Rejection Region}_j}^{\infty}\left[\prod_{i=1}^{Nj} f_{\theta_1}(x_i)\right]\cdot dx_1 \ldots dx_{N_j}}{\displaystyle\int_{\text{Rejection Region}_j}^{\infty}\left[\prod_{i=1}^{Nj} f_{\theta_0}(x_i)\right]\cdot dx_1 \ldots dx_{N_j}} > r \qquad (11.4)$$

at each analysis j. Now if the change in power divided by the change in type 1 error is greater than r at each analysis, then the cumulative power divided by the cumulative type 1 error is greater than r as well. Thus, the likelihood ratio test is a natural test to apply to ensure that the evidence in favor of the alternative conditional on when the study stopped exceeds a predefined constant.

11.2 Pocock Boundary

Another boundary that is often used in clinical trials is the Pocock boundary. The Pocock boundary rejects the null hypothesis at each analysis using the same critical value on the Z scale. Table 11.1 presents the operating characteristics for a Pocock rejection boundary. Whereas the O'Brien-Fleming boundary starts out with a ratio of power to type error that is much greater than 32, we can see in Table 11.1 that the Pocock boundary starts out with a ratio of power to type 1 error at the first analysis that is less than 32 and gradually increases to 32 from the first analysis to the last analysis. In Figure 11.1, we see that the ratio of the change in power to the change in type

TABLE 11.1

Summary of Power and Type 1 Error for a Pocock Boundary

	Interim 1	Interim 2	Interim 3	Interim 4	Interim 5	Interim 6	Final Analysis
Number of subjects per group	14	29	43	57	71	86	100
Z-statistic	2.49	2.49	2.49	2.49	2.49	2.49	2.49
Cumulative power	0.098	0.238	0.384	0.518	0.633	0.726	0.8
Cumulative type 1 error (one-sided)	0.006	0.011	0.015	0.018	0.021	0.023	0.025
β/α	16.33	21.64	25.6	28.78	30.14	31.57	32
$\Delta\beta/\Delta\alpha$	—	28	36.5	44.67	38.33	46.5	37
Effect size	0.315						

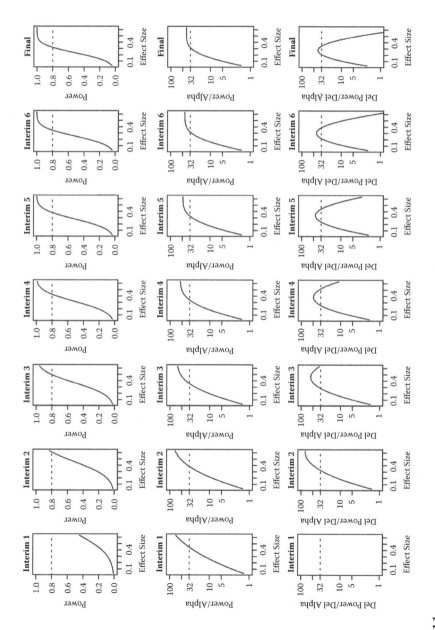

FIGURE 11.1
Operating characteristics of a Pocock boundary.

1 error is always greater than 32 for some treatment effect size. The Pocock boundary differs in this regard from the O'Brien-Fleming boundary we evaluated in Table 10.3 where the ratio of the change in power to the change in type 1 error was less than 32 at the final analysis for all treatment effect sizes. So, while one should be concerned about a study that rejects at the last analysis of an O'Brien-Fleming stopping boundary, one should also be concerned about a study that stops at the first analysis of a Pocock boundary. In this situation, there are clinically meaningful alternatives that have a low ratio of power to type 1 error and hence rejecting the null hypothesis by the Pocock boundary at an early analysis may lead to the regulator and society assuming more risk than desired.

References

Pocock, S.J. 1977. Group sequential methods in the design and analysis of clinical trials. *Biometrika* 64(2):191–199.

Wald, A. 1947. *Sequential Analysis.* New York: John Wiley.

12

Confirmatory Trials

A British television show featuring a magician carried an episode where the magician claimed to have a system for picking the winning horses at the racetrack. The show focused on a woman who received the magician's picks for the winning horses in each of five races. All five horses the magician picked for her did go on to win their respective races. The predictions were made at least 24 hours in advance of each race and the five races were spread over the course of a month. After receiving these tips, the woman was convinced that the magician could pick the winning horses at the track and was ready to bet all her money and money that her friends and relatives had loaned her on the next horse the magician picked to win its race.

The show then went on to reveal to this woman and the audience that she was not the only person who received the tips for the winning horses at the racetrack. There were many others who received predictions as well. However, for all but the woman the show focused on, at least one of the five tips for the winning horses was wrong. The magician had sent out tips for the winning horses to as many people as there were possible guesses for the winning horses in five races, $4^5 = 1024$. The woman who received the winning predictions for all five races was just 1 of these 1024 people. So, even though it appeared to the woman that the magician could predict the winning horses at the track, in fact the multiple guesses guaranteed that he would be correct at least once in predicting the winning horses in five races. No special ability on the part of the magician was required. Looking at all that the magician did revealed he was no better at predicting winning horses than anyone else.

This horse racing story is an example of how the context in which an event is evaluated can dramatically alter its perceived probability of occurrence. From the woman's point of view, it was highly unlikely that the magician could pick the winning horse in five consecutive races. Indeed, the probability of picking the winning horse for each of five consecutive races with four horses in each race is $0.25^5 \approx 0.001$. However, from the magician's perspective, he was certain that one person would receive five correct predictions for the winning horses at the track since as many unique individuals received predictions for the winning horses as there were unique possible combinations of horses winning the five races.

A positive Phase 2 trial can also be viewed in two different contexts that are similar to how the woman and the magician viewed the five correct predictions for the horse races. From the perspective of the sponsor of a positive

Phase 2 trial, statistically significant Phase 2 results are unlikely due to chance and consequently are deserving of serious consideration as evidence of the drug's effectiveness by regulatory agencies. This view parallels the view of the woman who received the horse racing tips from the magician. However, from the perspective of a regulatory agency, a positive Phase 2 trial is just one of many Phase 2 trials that are undertaken, one of which is almost guaranteed to be positive even if none of the drugs that are studied are effective. Indeed, the probability under the null hypothesis that at least 1 of 30 Phase 2 trials is significant at the 0.10 level is 0.957. This view of a positive Phase 2 trial parallels the magician's view of his horse racing predictions in which he was certain at least one person would receive five correct predictions for the winning horses at the track.

It should be further noted that a positive Phase 3 trial could be viewed in these two different contexts as well, although one would have to be more pessimistic about the quality of the drug development process than in the case of a positive Phase 2 trial.

In one of the horse races where the magician "predicted" the winner, the horse that was the favorite to win was leading the race from the start until it stumbled and was not able to get up. Following the accident, the horse that the magician had picked to win went into the lead and subsequently won the race. If the woman who received the five correct tips from the magician had thought to herself, "It isn't possible to predict that a horse will fall down in a race" and then went on to ask the magician to predict some more races, she would have learned that the magician in fact was not able to predict the winning horses. Similarly, in the development of new drugs, companies are asked to replicate the promising results seen in Phase 2 by running Phase 3 "confirmatory" trials. Oftentimes, these Phase 3 trials do not result in the same encouraging results seen in Phase 2, sparing the public from the costs of using ineffective drugs. In addition, sometimes a single Phase 3 trial is not considered enough evidence to support registration and a second Phase 3 trial may be requested. The need to distinguish between positive Phase 2 and Phase 3 results that are due to chance and those that are due to an active drug is why confirmatory trials are part of the drug development process. In other words, confirmation is concerned with ruling out that positive study results are explainable under a global null hypothesis.

In this chapter we will take a look at two issues in clinical trials that are tied to whether study results are consistent with the global null hypothesis. The first issue we will address is whether Phase 2 data can be combined with data from Phase 3 trials. That is, can we combine results from Phase 2 and Phase 3 to reduce the total number of subjects required to achieve a significant p-value with sufficient power that will support regulatory approval. The second issue we will address is whether a single Phase 3 trial can be considered confirmatory. That is, can we rule out that a positive Phase 3 trial is consistent with the global null hypothesis without performing a second Phase 3 trial. First, we will address combining data from Phase 2 and Phase 3.

12.1 Can Evidence from Phase 2 Trials Be Combined with Evidence from Phase 3?

Phase 2 trials of new drug candidates are generally not considered to provide confirmatory evidence of a drug's effectiveness because they are undertaken in great numbers and most of these studies turn out negative. That is, a Phase 2 trial is not confirmatory because it can be considered as one of many similar but failed trials. When the results of a positive Phase 2 trial are considered in the light of all the other similar negative trials that were conducted, the statistical significance of the result is much less certain and the need for a follow-up confirmatory trial becomes clear.

To formally address the question of whether a Phase 2 trial can be pooled with a Phase 3 confirmatory trial, consider a study design with an interim analysis plan that includes one futility analysis that is conducted at an intermediate point of the study followed by the final analysis. A Phase 2 trial followed by a Phase 3 trial can be viewed as a special case of this design where the trial prior to the interim futility analysis can be thought of as a Phase 2 study, whereas the portion of the trial that follows the futility analysis can be thought of as the Phase 3 study. We will be looking at the design this way for the purpose of evaluating the poolability of Phase 2 and Phase 3 studies.

The type 1 error for this trial is the probability that it will not stop for futility and will be positive at the final analysis under the null hypothesis that the treatment under investigation has no effect. We will denote this probability by $P_{\theta_0}(+)$. The probability model that is used in this calculation of the type 1 error only considers outcomes of the study and so accurately reflects the significance of the results from the point of view of the experimenter.

Now consider the results of the trial from the perspective of a reviewer who has to recommend whether to grant marketing approval. For studies like the one described here, the reviewer will never make a decision regarding marketing approval when the study stops at the interim futility analysis. That is, the reviewer is only asked to consider studies that stopped at the final analysis. Thus, the probability of a positive result under the null hypothesis for all studies that continue to the final analysis is a more relevant error probability for the reviewer's decision making than the probability of a positive result for the study as a whole. This probability will be denoted as $P_{\theta_0}(+ \mid \text{Stop at Final Analysis})$.

Now the type 1 error from the perspective of the experimenter can be related to the type 1 error from the perspective of the reviewer by the expression

$$P_{\theta_0}(+) = \sum_{t_i} P_{\theta_0}(+, \text{ Stop at } t_i) = \sum_{t_i} P_{\theta_0}(\text{Stop at } t_i) \cdot P_{\theta_0}(+ \mid \text{Stop at } t_i) \quad (12.1)$$

The key quantities that relate the viewpoint of the experimenter with the viewpoint of the reviewer are $P_{\theta_0}\left(\text{Stop at } t_i\right)$. From the experimenter's point of view, $P_{\theta_0}\left(\text{Stop at } t_i\right)$ is simply the probability of the study stopping at analysis i if the data collected in the study follow the distribution assumed under the null hypothesis. However, a reviewer looking at the positive results of a study that continued to the final analysis will never consider the results of those studies that stopped early for futility. So, in the sample space of studies that the reviewer is asked to consider, the reviewer treats the probability of stopping at t_1 as 0

$$P_{\theta_0}\left(\text{Stop at } t_1\right) = 0 \qquad (12.2)$$

and the probability of stopping at t_2 as

$$P_{\theta_0}\left(\text{Stop at } t_2\right) = 1 \qquad (12.3)$$

and so the probability of a type 1 error for the reviewer is

$$P_{\theta_0}\left(+\right) = P_{\theta_0}\left(+ \,|\, \text{Stop at } t_2\right) \qquad (12.4)$$

As an example, let's consider the following very simple interim analysis plan presented in Table 12.1. In this interim analysis plan, the total type 1 error as would be reported by the experimenter is 0.0206 (0.025 if we ignore the futility boundary). However, as considered by a reviewer who is interested in the results conditional on the study making it to the end, the probability of seeing a positive result under the null hypothesis is

$$\frac{0.0206 - 0.0026}{1 - 0.8413} = 0.1134 \qquad (12.5)$$

TABLE 12.1

Summary of Power and Type 1 Error for a Study with a Single Interim Analysis

	Interim 1	Final Analysis
Total number of events	224	447
Z-statistic (reject the null)	2.796	1.977
Z-statistic (reject the alt)	1	1.977
Cumulative power	0.26	0.8015
Cumulative type 1 error (one-sided)	0.0026	0.0206
Cumulative probability of stopping for futility (alt)	0.1245	0.1985
Cumulative probability of stopping for futility (null)	0.8413	0.9794
Post probability alt true given no stopping	0.8	NA
Ratio of beta to alpha	100.49	39
Delta power/Delta alpha	—	30.14
Effect size	0.75	

This represents an important discrepancy between how the experimenter and the reviewer interpret the results of a positive study.

Now the experimenter would argue the probability under the null hypothesis that the study would stop at the last analysis is very small, 0.16, and so the type 1 error that the reviewer is using is too large. However, from the reviewer's perspective, it could be argued that the probability a study stops at the last analysis also depends on all the other similar studies that have been performed. The probability model for the reviewer's evaluation of the null hypothesis may be called the global null and is generated by a process where consecutive studies with a similar design to the one at hand evaluate treatments with no effect. Note that the probability model for the global null hypothesis corresponds to the model used for evaluating efficiency with $p = 0$. In this view there are sufficient replications of similar trials that a study that does not stop at the interim analysis will be generated with probability one even when all the trials represent a drug with no activity.

The perspectives of the experimenter and the reviewer as just described are polar opposites. In the view of the experimenter, there is only one study that contributes to the calculation of $P_{\theta_0}\left(\text{Stop at } t_1\right)$, whereas in the view of the reviewer there are an untold number of studies that can contribute to its determination. What about intermediate circumstances? Table 12.2 presents the probability that the Phase 2 portion of the study is not positive along with the statistical significance of the study as a whole under the global null where the number of Phase 2 studies that can contribute to the calculation of $P_{\theta_0}\left(\text{Stop at } t_1\right)$ ranges from 1 to 40. We arbitrarily picked $Z > 1$ as the significance level that makes the Phase 2 positive to be consistent with the example presented in Table 12.1. Now in Table 12.2 we see, for example, that if the reviewer believes there are 10 similar Phase 2 studies that can be considered together with the study at hand, either because they were in the same patient population or the same time period, then under the global null hypothesis that none of the drugs studied are effective the type 1 error for the study at hand would be 0.093.

TABLE 12.2

Probability of a Type 1 Error under the Global Null Hypothesis

Number of Studies (n)	P(Stop at Futility Analysis) $P_{\theta_0}\left(n/n \text{ studies stop at } t_1\right)$	Type 1 Error $\left[1 - P_{\theta_0}\left(n/n \text{ studies stop at } t_1\right)\right] \cdot P_{\theta_0}\left(+ \,\vert\, \text{Stop at } t_2\right)$
1	0.841	0.018
2	0.708	0.033
5	0.422	0.066
10	0.178	0.093
20	0.032	0.110
40	0.001	0.113

Now let's suppose that among these 10 Phase 2 studies the reviewer identified, we know that 2 of them had positive results in the sense that the Z-statistic for the primary endpoint was greater than 1. In this case the probability of moving past the first stage of the trial could be viewed as the probability of moving past the first stage in at least 2 of 10 studies. As such, the probability of a type 1 error for this study would be

$$P_{\theta_0}(\geq 2/10 + \text{Phase 2 Trials}) \cdot P_{\theta_0}(+\,|\,\text{Stop at } t_2) = 0.4871 \times 0.1134 = 0.0553 \quad (12.6)$$

With three positive Phase 2 trials we have

$$P_{\theta_0}(\geq 3/10 + \text{Phase 2 Trials}) \cdot P_{\theta_0}(+\,|\,\text{Stop at } t_2) = 0.2028 \times 0.1134 = 0.0230 \quad (12.7)$$

Whereas if 4 of these 10 studies were positive, then the type 1 error under the global null would be

$$P_{\theta_0}(\geq 4/10 + \text{Phase 2 Trials}) \cdot P_{\theta_0}(+\,|\,\text{Stop at } t_2) = 0.0597 \times 0.1134 = 0.0067 \quad (12.8)$$

So, if the evidence in a collection of similar Phase 2 studies suggests that the global null hypothesis is not true, as in the case where 3 of 10 or 4 of 10 Phase 2 trials are positive, then the type 1 error from the perspective of the reviewer may actually be less than the type 1 error from the perspective of the experimenter, in which case the results from Phase 2 and Phase 3 can be pooled together without having to worry about the *p*-value being compromised by the global null hypothesis. Now the number of events required to have 80 percent power to detect a hazard ratio of 0.75 is 382. Thus, by pooling the Phase 2 and Phase 3 data in this example, instead of observing 224 + 382 = 606 events one would only have to observe 447 events to have an 80 percent chance of observing a statistically significant result after completing Phase 2 and Phase 3, a savings of 159 events.

12.2 Example: Phase 2 in Rheumatoid Arthritis

Here we consider whether the Phase 2 and Phase 3 studies in a clinical program for rheumatoid arthritis could be combined without having to worry about the *p*-value being corrupted by the global null hypothesis. Table 12.3 presents the Phase 2 industry sponsored studies in rheumatoid arthritis that

TABLE 12.3

Results from Phase 2 Trials in Rheumatoid Arthritis: January 1, 2001–January 1, 2005

Drug	Phase 2 Result	Positive	Source
AMG-719	Unknown	–	
Belimumab	Improved ACR20, not ACR50 or 70; more work to identify patient population	+	A safety and efficacy study of LymphoStat-B™ (monoclonal anti-BLyS antibody) in subjects with rheumatoid arthritis (RA), www.clinicaltrials.gov, NCT00071812
CCI-779	Unknown	–	
Denosumab	$P = 0.019$	+	Cohen, S.B., et al., 2008, Denosumab treatment effects on structural damage, bone mineral density, and bone turnover in rheumatoid arthritis: A twelve-month, multicenter, randomized, double-blind, placebo-controlled, phase II clinical trial, *Arthritis and Rheumatism* 58(5):1299–1309.
Efalizumab	No net clinical benefit	–	Eustice, C., 2009, Raptiva (efalizumab) drug trial halted, http://arthritis.about.com/cs/druggen/a/raptiva.htm
HuMax-CD4	No sig diff in ACR scores	–	http://www.docguide.com/humax-cd4-combination-therapy-not-effective-rheumatoid-arthritis
ISIS-104838	$P = 0.04$	+	http://ir.isispharm.com/phoenix.zhtml?c=222170&p=irol-newsArticle_pf&ID=1289726&highlight
Medi-522 (Vitaxin)	No clinical benefit	–	MEDI 522 MedImmune discontinued, 2004, http://business.highbeam.com/436989/article-1G1-121568456/medi-522
Natalizumab	$P = 0.089$	+	Natalizumab in the treatment of rheumatoid arthritis in subjects receiving methotrexate, Clinicaltrials.gov, NCT00083759
Ocrelizumab	$P < 0.01$	+	Genovese, M.C., et al., 2008, Ocrelizumab, a humanized anti-CD20 monoclonal antibody, in the treatment of patients with rheumatoid arthritis: A phase I/II randomized, blinded, placebo-controlled, dose-ranging study, *Arthritis and Rheumatism* 58(9):2652–2661
Paxceed	Unknown	–	
SCIO469	$P = 0.583$	–	Bonilla-Hernán, M.G., et al., 2011, New drugs beyond biologics in rheumatoid arthritis: The kinase inhibitors, *Rheumatology* 50(9):1542–1550.
TMI-005	Negative	–	Moss, M.L., et al., 2008. Drug Insight: Tumor necrosis factor converting enzyme as a pharmaceutical target for rheumatoid arthritis. *Nature Clinical Practice Rheumatology* 4(6):300–309

were undertaken in the period from January 1, 2001 to January 1, 2005, as determined by www.clinicaltrials.gov.

Five of these 12 clinical trials reported some sort of positive results. The probability of seeing 5 or more of 12 clinical trials with positive results ($Z > 1$) when the treatments are not effective is 0.0300, whereas the probability that a single trial will have such a positive result is 0.1587. Thus, we could conclude in these circumstances that the Phase 2 and Phase 3 studies from a clinical trial program can be combined, provided of course that the patient population and doses administered are the same.

12.3 Design a Phase 3 Trial to Account for Evidence against the Global Null Hypothesis

Let's continue our discussion of the situation where the reviewer has identified 10 Phase 2 trials that are similar to the study under consideration. And let's further suppose that just 2 of these 10 Phase 2 trials are positive. What would the Phase 3 trial have to look like to make the data from the combined Phase 2 and Phase 3 phases of clinical development statistically significant under the global null?

The type 1 error would have to be such that

$$P_{\theta_0}(\geq 2/10 + \text{Phase 2 Trials}) \cdot P_{\theta_0}(+\,|\,\text{Stop at } t_2) = 0.4871 \times \frac{\alpha_3 - 0.0026}{1 - 0.8413} = 0.025 \tag{12.9}$$

and so

$$\alpha_3 = 0.025 \times (1 - 0.8413) + 0.0026 = 0.0107 \tag{12.10}$$

Making use of the calculation in Equation (12.10) for the type 1 error, Table 12.4 presents a Phase 2/Phase 3 study design that is statistically significant under the global null if at least 2 out of the 10 similar Phase 2 studies are positive. By keeping the first part of the trial as before, enlarging the total number of events from 447 to 551 and by testing at the final analysis with $Z = 2.285$ the trial becomes statistically significant under the global as well as the standard null hypothesis. In this situation, a total of 55 events (($224 + 382$) $- 551 = 55$) could be saved by pooling Phase 2 with Phase 3.

Recall that in the previous example, we arbitrarily set the criteria for stopping for futility at the end of Phase 2 as $Z > 1$. If the Z-value for stopping for futility is made more strict, for example, $Z > 1.5$ or $Z > 1$ at 100 events instead of 224 events, at some point the power for the combined Phase 2/Phase 3 trial will necessarily decrease regardless of the number of subjects in

TABLE 12.4

Study Design That Leads to Statistical Significance under the Global Null
Hypothesis When 2 of 10 Phase 2 Studies Are Positive (Z > 1)

	Interim 1	Final Analysis
Total number of events	224	551
Z-statistic (reject the null)	2.796	2.285
Z-statistic (reject the alt)	1	2.285
Cumulative power	0.26	0.8001
Cumulative type 1 error (one-sided)	0.0026	0.0106
Cumulative probability of stopping for futility (alt)	0.1245	0.1999
Cumulative probability of stopping for futility (null)	0.8413	0.9894
Post prob alt true given no stopping	0.8	NA
Ratio of beta to alpha	100.52	75.2
del power/del alpha	0	67.06
Effect size	0.75	

the Phase 3 portion of the trial because the test for futility at the end of Phase 2 reduces the number of sample paths that can lead to rejection of the null for the combined Phase 2 and Phase 3 study. So, for example, if the probability of stopping for futility under the alternative at the end of the Phase 2 portion of the trial is greater than 0.20, then it is impossible for the combined Phase 2/3 trial to have power of 80 percent or more. On the other hand, if the z-value is not strict, meaning that Phase 3 may be initiated even without a positive Phase 2, then the power of the combined trial will not carry such a restriction. Unfortunately, the criteria a company uses to start a Phase 3 trial based on Phase 2 data is usually not specified completely in advance of the decision. So a regulator would be forced to take the worst-case scenario since the burden of proving a drug works lies with the sponsor. That is, the regulator would be forced to assume that the Phase 2 rejection boundary was at least as strict as the data that was observed and therefore, depending on the observed Phase 2 result, the power of the combined data set may be low. Thus, obtaining a sufficiently powered "Phase 3" trial by combining Phase 2 data and Phase 3 data may not be so easy unless the Phase 2 trial is not used as a screening trial and is truly used just to fine-tune the Phase 3 design.

Now we switch perspectives and consider how combining the data from the Phase 2 and Phase 3 trials impacts the strength of evidence in favor of marketing approval as compared with simply treating them as separate trials using Power/Type 1 error as the measure of evidence. Table 12.5 presents the ratio of power to type 1 error calculated when the Phase 2 and Phase 3 trials are considered separately as well as when they are considered to be one trial.

In Table 12.5, $\alpha_{Futility}$ represents the significance level for the futility boundary at the end of Phase 2 and α_3 represents the type 1 error at the final analysis in Phase 3. The power of the combined Phase 2 and Phase 3 trials (column 6) represents the power of the combined analysis after accounting

TABLE 12.5

Ratio of Power to Type 1 Error as a Function of the Phase 2 Sample Size and Futility Boundary

$N_{Phase\,2}$	$\alpha_{Futility}$	$N_{Phase\,3}$	$N_{Phase\,2} + N_{Phase\,3}$	α_3	Power of Combined Phase 2 and Phase 3	β/α				
						Phase 2	Phase 3	Phase 2 and Phase 3 Separate	Phase 2 and Phase 3 Separate; 80% Power Phase 3	Phase 2 and Phase 3 Combined
50	0.9	335	385	0.024	0.801	1.1	30.0	33.0	35.2	33.4
50	0.7	371	421	0.022	0.801	1.3	31.6	42.4	42.9	36.4
50	0.5	529	579	0.018	0.801	1.7	36.4	61.6	54.1	44.5
50	0.3	800	850	0.013	0.684	2.3	39.3	90.2	73.5	52.6
50	0.1	800	850	0.006	0.394	4.0	39.3	155.5	126.6	65.7
100	0.9	281	381	0.025	0.801	1.1	27.0	29.9	35.4	32.0
100	0.7	289	389	0.023	0.801	1.4	27.5	38.2	44.6	34.8
100	0.5	323	423	0.020	0.801	1.8	29.4	54.3	59.2	40.1
100	0.3	578	678	0.015	0.801	2.7	37.3	102.0	87.4	53.4
100	0.1	800	900	0.007	0.561	5.6	39.3	221.0	179.9	80.1
150	0.9	230	380	0.025	0.801	1.1	23.5	26.1	35.5	32.0
150	0.7	232	382	0.024	0.801	1.4	23.7	33.4	45.2	33.4
150	0.5	241	391	0.021	0.801	1.9	24.3	46.7	61.5	38.1
150	0.3	295	445	0.017	0.801	3.0	27.8	82.7	95.1	47.1
150	0.1	800	950	0.009	0.684	6.8	39.3	269.0	219.0	76.0

for the futility boundary that describes the Phase 2 go/no–go decision. β/α Phase 2 represents the ratio of power to type 1 error in the Phase 2 trial, β/α Phase 3 represents the ratio of power to type 1 error in the Phase 3 trial, β/α Phase 2 and 3 separate represents the products of β/α Phase 2 and β/α Phase 3. β/α Phase 2 and 3 separate–power 80 percent represents the ratio of power to type 1 error when the Phase 2 and Phase 3 trials are treated separately and the Phase 3 trials is powered at 80 percent. And finally, β/α Phase 2 and 3 combined represents the ratio of power to type 1 error when the Phase 2 and Phase 3 trials are combined.

Table 12.5 shows that with a Phase 2 sample size of 50 per group and a futility boundary associated with an alpha level of 0.9, there is very little difference between the ratio of power to type 1 error whether one combines the Phase 2 and Phase 3 studies in which case the ratio of power to type 1 error is 33.4 or whether one treats them as separate studies, which results in a ratio of power to type 1 error of 33.0. On the other hand, as the futility boundary becomes stricter and the associated alpha level decreases from 0.9 to 0.1, the ratio of power to type 1 error increases much more in the situation where the Phase 2 and Phase 3 studies are treated separately than when they are combined. Indeed, at a futility boundary corresponding to an alpha level of 0.10 one-sided we see that the ratio of power to type 1 error when the Phase 2 and Phase 3 studies are treated separately and Phase 3 is powerd at 80 percent is 127. This compares with a ratio of 66 when the studies are pooled together. Clearly then, there is a large advantage in terms of the ratio of power to type 1 error and ultimately the ratio of true to false positives to treating the Phase 2 and Phase 3 trials separately when the Phase 2 trial is used as a screening trial to determine whether Phase 3 is undertaken.

Another interesting item to note in Table 12.5 is that when the alpha level for futility is quite low the number of subjects required to have 80 percent power when the Phase 2 and Phase 3 studies are combined is higher than when the Phase 2 and Phase 3 trials are treated separately. For example, when $\alpha_{Futility} = 0.9$, the total number of subjects required in Phase 2 and 3 to attain 80 percent power is 385. However, when $\alpha_{Futility} = 0.1$, 850 subjects in Phase 2 and Phase 3 combined provides only 39.4 percent power. This is what we expected to see since as we noted earlier a strict futility boundary at the end of Phase 2 reduces the number of sample paths that can result in a positive Phase 3 trial.

12.4 Evidence from Phase 3 Trials

A confirmatory trial is a Phase 3 trial that establishes that a drug has clinical benefit following completion of testing in Phase 2. There are many features of a Phase 3 clinical trial that make it confirmatory. The primary hypothesis has to be well specified, the population to be studied must be clearly identified, and the method of testing has to be specified *a priori*. All of these features help to ensure that the probability of a positive result under the null hypothesis is not inflated above the prespecified level of significance. In addition to all these requirements and perhaps most important, a confirmatory trial must not be conducted under circumstances similar to what the lady in the horse racing example found herself in. That is, a confirmatory trial cannot be viewed as one of many other similar but failed studies. If a confirmatory trial can be viewed as such, then a positive result may simply be due to chance rather than the experimental treatment just as the winning horse predictions the woman received were not evidence that the magician had a special talent for picking the winning horses at the races.

In some situations, a single Phase 3 trial is deemed enough information for marketing approval, whereas in other cases two Phase 3 studies are required. The criteria used in practice for deciding when to require two studies are based primarily on medical need. If there is a great medical need then only one trial will be required, whereas if there is not such a great medical need, as in the case of the second drug in a new class, two studies will be required. Here, we try to develop criteria for when one or two trials are required based on the level of evidence produced by clinical trials.

Suppose a reviewer is looking at the results of a positive Phase 3 trial and wants to discern between study results that are due to an active drug and those that are due to chance. The probability space that this reviewer faces is one in which the Phase 3 trial is always positive. Thus, the statistical significance of the study under consideration is not informative and the reviewer needs to look at the success rate of other similar trials to judge whether the drug development process is generating true positive or false positive Phase 3 trials. Suppose, for example, that two of the last four Phase 3 trials in lung cancer, not including the current one under consideration, were statistically significant at the 0.025 level of significance. The probability that two or more out of four Phase 3 confirmatory trials would be positive simply due to chance is

$$\sum_{i=2}^{4} \binom{4}{i} \cdot 0.025^i \cdot 0.975^{4-i} = 0.0036 \tag{12.11}$$

So, in these circumstances we could say that the recent history of drug development in lung cancer provides enough evidence to reject the global null hypothesis that positive Phase 3 lung cancer trials are all simply due to chance. On the other hand, if three of the previous four trials were negative and one was positive, the probability of seeing one or more positive trials under the global null hypothesis would be 0.09630. This would not be enough evidence to disprove the hypothesis that positive Phase 3 trials are due solely to chance. In this circumstance, one would necessarily have to conduct a second Phase 3 trial to provide enough evidence that the first positive Phase 3 trial is not simply an artifact of repeated Phase 3 trials where the molecule under study is not effective.

A significant p-value for a test of the global null hypothesis is not enough evidence to permit a drug to be approved based on a single Phase 3 trial. The power to detect a reasonable alternative with an acceptable ratio of true to false positives is also important. If that power is too low, then the strength of evidence against the global null may not be sufficient.

To calculate this power we will use the model presented and developed in earlier chapters to evaluate the efficiency of drug development. We will also make the simplifying assumption for the purposes of this power calculation that the drug development programs included in the analysis use similar designs for Phase 2 and Phase 3. The proportion of initiated Phase 3 trials that are positive can be expressed as

$$\pi = \frac{p \cdot \Phi\left(z_{\alpha_2} - (z_{\alpha_3} - z_\beta) \cdot f_\delta \sqrt{f_N}\right) \cdot \Phi\left(z_{\alpha_3} - (z_{\alpha_3} - z_\beta) \cdot f_\delta\right) + (1-p) \cdot \alpha_2 \cdot \alpha_3}{p \cdot \Phi\left(z_{\alpha_2} - (z_{\alpha_3} - z_\beta) \cdot f_\delta \sqrt{f_N}\right) + (1-p) \cdot \alpha_2} \tag{12.12}$$

The probability that more than k Phase 3 trials will be positive out of N initiated Phase 3 trials will then be

$$\sum_{i=k}^{N} \binom{N}{i} \pi^i (1-\pi)^{N-i} \tag{12.13}$$

The larger π is, the fewer number of studies required to reject the global null hypothesis. The ratio π is affected by the rate of effective drugs going into development, p, as well as z_{α_2}, the critical value for evaluating Phase 2 trials. The stricter the z-value for evaluating Phase 2, the greater the proportion of Phase 3 trials that will be positive.

Although π is important for determining the power to reject the global null hypothesis, the ratio of true to false positives ultimately determines the quality of the decision to grant marketing approval to a drug. The ratio of true to false positives can be expressed as

$$\frac{T+}{F+} = \frac{p \cdot \Phi\left(z_{\alpha_2} - (z_{\alpha_3} - z_\beta) \cdot f_\delta \sqrt{f_N}\right) \cdot \Phi\left(z_{\alpha_3} - (z_{\alpha_3} - z_\beta) \cdot f_\delta\right)}{(1-p) \cdot \alpha_2 \cdot \alpha_3} \tag{12.14}$$

This expression shows that the relative numbers of true and false positive Phase 3 trials depends on the proportion of molecules entering the drug development process that do have some clinical benefit as well as the design of the Phase 2 and Phase 3 trials. Given the designs of the Phase 2 and Phase 3 trials as well as the ratio of true to false positives that we wish to detect, one can assess whether there will be enough power to reject the global null.

Figure 12.1 presents the power to reject the global null for a range of values for α_2 and f_N when the results of Phase 3 trials from 10 drug development programs are available. In addition to the power, Figure 12.1 also presents the proportion of Phase 3 trials that would be expected to be positive along with the ratio of true to false positives. The calculations assume that $p = 0.10$ and $f_8 = 1$.

Figure 12.1 shows that the greater the sample size in Phase 2 the greater the proportion of Phase 3 trials that are positive and *a fortiori* the power to reject the global null hypothesis. In addition, the ratio of true to false positives also increases as the Phase 2 sample size increases. Similarly, as α_2 decreases, the power, proportion of positive Phase 3 trials, and the ratio of true to false positives all increase.

The third row of Figure 12.1 presents the ratio of true to false positives. The ratio of true to false positives may be as low as three when the efficacy results from the Phase 2 trial are not used as a gate for starting Phase 3, that is when $\alpha_2 = 0.99$. With z values that are stricter the ratio of true to false positives can be increased. For example, an α_2 level of 0.05 with a Phase 2 sample size of $f_N = 0.20$ would result in a ratio of true to false positives of 25.

Table 12.6 is a tabular presentation of the results in Figure 12.1 with the additional cases where $p = 0.20$ and $p = 0.30$. Table 12.6 shows that the higher the probability, p, that the drug will provide clinical benefit at the outset of Phase 2, the greater the power, the proportion of Phase 3 trials that are positive, and the ratio of true positives to false positives.

As noted earlier, the ratio of true to false positives is dependent on the study designs in Phase 2 and Phase 3, the decision criteria used to move a molecule to Phase 3, and the rate at which effective drugs enter clinical development. If we knew all these factors we could estimate the ratio of true to false positives for a particular development program. Although the factors affecting the ratio of true to false positives related to the study designs are relatively easy to get, determining the rate at which effective drugs enter clinical development is more challenging. It requires the analysis of historical data concerning Phase 2 and Phase 3 trials across many compounds.

An example of such historical data is provided by Chan et al. (2008), who presented an analysis of Phase 2 studies and subsequent Phase 3 trials that focused on evaluating the factors in Phase 2 that were predictive of success in Phase 3. They looked at approximately 300 Phase 3 trials and their precedent Phase 2 trials. Although such a data set can be used to estimate the impact of Phase 2 characteristics on the Phase 3 success rate, it cannot be used to estimate the proportion of molecules entering drug development that can provide a clinical benefit. The main reason is that not all Phase 2 trials are followed by a Phase 3 trial and the exact criteria by which it is decided to start Phase 3 is not always known. Fortunately, regulatory agencies are in a position to know the results of Phase 2 trials that are not followed up with Phase 3 trials. If the data set used by Chan et al. is expanded

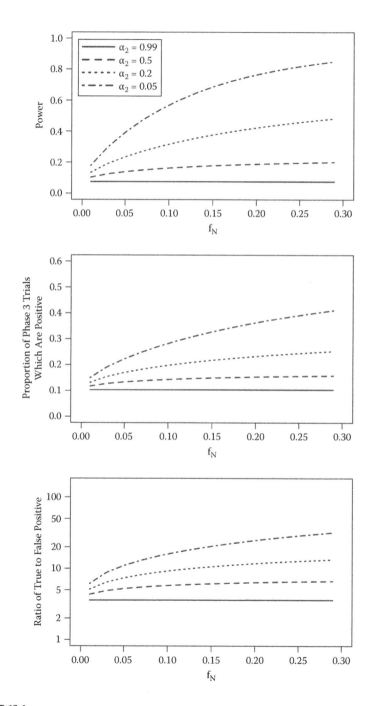

FIGURE 12.1
Power to detect that positive Phase 3 trials are not simply due to chance with the results of ten
Phase 3 trials. $p = 0.1$ and $f_\delta = 1$.

TABLE 12.6

Power to Reject the Global Null, Proportion of Phase 3 Trials That Are Positive, and the Ratio for True Positives to False Positives

f_δ	p	$z_{\alpha 2}$	f_N	Proportion of Phase 3 Trials That Are Positive	Power to Reject the Global Null with Five Phase 3 Trials[a]	Error in Rejecting the Global Null with Five Phase 3 Trials[a]	Power to Reject the Global Null with Ten Phase 3 Trials[b]	Error in Rejecting the Global Null with Ten Phase 3 Trials[b]	Ratio of True Positives to False Positives
1	0.1	0.99	0.1	0.103	0.086	0.006	0.076	0.002	3.589
1	0.1	0.99	0.2	0.103	0.086	0.006	0.076	0.002	3.591
1	0.1	0.99	0.3	0.103	0.086	0.006	0.076	0.002	3.591
1	0.1	0.50	0.1	0.143	0.153	0.006	0.163	0.002	5.775
1	0.1	0.50	0.2	0.154	0.171	0.006	0.189	0.002	6.364
1	0.1	0.50	0.3	0.159	0.181	0.006	0.203	0.002	6.667
1	0.1	0.20	0.1	0.198	0.259	0.006	0.316	0.002	9.203
1	0.1	0.20	0.2	0.233	0.331	0.006	0.422	0.002	11.726
1	0.1	0.20	0.3	0.254	0.376	0.006	0.487	0.002	13.437
1	0.1	0.05	0.1	0.283	0.436	0.006	0.569	0.002	15.925
1	0.1	0.05	0.2	0.363	0.596	0.006	0.765	0.002	24.715
1	0.1	0.05	0.3	0.415	0.689	0.006	0.856	0.002	32.431
1	0.2	0.99	0.1	0.181	0.225	0.006	0.266	0.002	8.075
1	0.2	0.99	0.2	0.181	0.225	0.006	0.266	0.002	8.079
1	0.2	0.99	0.3	0.181	0.225	0.006	0.266	0.002	8.080

1	0.2	0.50	0.1	0.249	0.365	0.006	0.471	0.002	12.995
1	0.2	0.50	0.2	0.265	0.398	0.006	0.518	0.002	14.318
1	0.2	0.50	0.3	0.272	0.414	0.006	0.540	0.002	15.001
1	0.2	0.20	0.1	0.329	0.531	0.006	0.692	0.002	20.707
1	0.2	0.20	0.2	0.375	0.619	0.006	0.789	0.002	26.383
1	0.2	0.20	0.3	0.401	0.666	0.006	0.835	0.002	30.232
1	0.2	0.05	0.1	0.434	0.720	0.006	0.882	0.002	35.832
1	0.2	0.05	0.2	0.517	0.833	0.006	0.956	0.002	55.608
1	0.2	0.05	0.3	0.564	0.882	0.006	0.978	0.002	72.970
1	0.3	0.99	0.1	0.259	0.386	0.006	0.501	0.002	13.844
1	0.3	0.99	0.2	0.259	0.386	0.006	0.502	0.002	13.850
1	0.3	0.99	0.3	0.259	0.386	0.006	0.502	0.002	13.852
1	0.3	0.50	0.1	0.343	0.558	0.006	0.723	0.002	22.277
1	0.3	0.50	0.2	0.361	0.593	0.006	0.762	0.002	24.545
1	0.3	0.50	0.3	0.370	0.610	0.006	0.780	0.002	25.716
1	0.3	0.20	0.1	0.433	0.717	0.006	0.880	0.002	35.498
1	0.3	0.20	0.2	0.479	0.785	0.006	0.929	0.002	45.228
1	0.3	0.20	0.3	0.504	0.818	0.006	0.948	0.002	51.827
1	0.3	0.05	0.1	0.535	0.853	0.006	0.966	0.002	61.427
1	0.3	0.05	0.2	0.605	0.917	0.006	0.989	0.002	95.328
1	0.3	0.05	0.3	0.642	0.941	0.006	0.994	0.002	125.091

[a] Reject if > 1 of 5 trials is significant.
[b] Reject if > 2 of 10 trials is significant.

to include the Phase 2 trials that are not followed by a Phase 3 trial, then we can estimate the probability a drug could provide clinical benefit. A simple estimate would be the proportion of all studies entering Phase 2 that ultimately are approved for marketing by a regulatory authority. This estimate would be expected to be smaller than the true rate but nonetheless provides us with a conservative starting point. Such estimates by clinical area are provided by DiMasi et al. (2010) for new molecules. We could also estimate the proportion of drugs that could provide benefit by maximum likelihood. This enables us to adjust our estimate of the probability that a drug that enters Phase 2 can provide a clinical benefit for the possibility that drugs for which Phase 3 trials are initiated have a higher likelihood of being successful.

If we let i index the molecules that were studied in Phase 2 and possibly Phase 3, then we can write the likelihood function for the collection of Phase 2 and Phase 3 trial results as

$$
L = \prod_{i=1}^{n} \left(\begin{array}{l} p^{\left(1-\hat{I}_{3,i}\right)} \cdot \left(p+p_s\right)^{\hat{I}_{3,i}} \cdot \phi_\sigma\left(z_{\alpha 2i} + \left[z_\beta - z_{\alpha 3i}\right] \cdot f_\delta \cdot \sqrt{f_{N,i}}\right) \\ \cdot \phi_\sigma\left(z_{\alpha 3i} + \left[z_\beta - z_{\alpha 3i}\right] \cdot f_\delta\right)^{\hat{I}_{3,i}} \\ + \left(1-p\right)^{\left(1-\hat{I}_{3,i}\right)} \cdot \left(1-p-p_s\right)^{\hat{I}_{3,i}} \cdot \phi\left(z_{\alpha 2i}\right) \cdot \phi\left(z_{\alpha 3i}\right)^{\hat{I}_{3,i}} \end{array} \right) \tag{12.15}
$$

Here, $\hat{I}_{3,i}$ is an indicator variable that is one if molecule i is studied in Phase 3 and zero otherwise. Note that if a molecule does not make it to Phase 3, then only the terms in Equation (12.15) related to the results in Phase 2 would be included in the portion of the likelihood function for that molecule. This model permits us to estimate the impact on the efficiency of drug development of scientifically interpreting the data collected in Phase 2, which is represented by the coefficient p_s, as well as the impact of using the Phase 2 trial as a screen, represented by the coefficients α_{2i} and $f_{N,i}$. The parameter σ represents a random effect on the treatment benefit observed across multiple molecules. The data to be collected to fit this model and the parameters to be estimated are described in Table 12.7.

With the maximum likelihood estimates and the information matrix derived from the aforementioned likelihood function, a confidence interval could be produced for the parameter p. With this analysis of historical data, we could make statements like we are x percent confident that the ratio of true to false positives is greater than y. If the estimate of p is sufficient to yield a ratio of true positives to false positives that is acceptable at a sufficient level of confidence, then a single Phase 3 trial may be deemed sufficient for marketing approval. Otherwise a second positive Phase 3 trial may be required.

TABLE 12.7

Data and Model Parameters for the Likelihood Function for Estimating p

Data	
$\hat{z}_{\alpha2,i}$	Z-statistic in Phase 2 for molecule i
$\hat{z}_{\alpha3,i}$	Z-statistic in Phase 3 for molecule i
$\hat{I}_{3,i}$	Indicator for whether Phase 3 trial for molecule i is initiated; 1 if Phase 3 initiated, 0 otherwise.
$f_{N2,i}$	Size of Phase 2 relative to standard Phase 3 trial for molecule i
$f_{N3,i}$	Size of Phase 3 relative to standard Phase 3 trial for molecule i
Parameters	
p_1	Underlying rate at which effective drugs enter clinical development
p_s	Increment in rate at which effective drugs enter clinical development arising from scientific interpretation of Phase 2 data
f_δ	The magnitude of the treatment effect relative to standard Phase 3 plan
σ	Random effect for treatment benefit in each study

It should be noted that the more complex the model is, the greater the number of observations required to get good estimates of the parameters. To attain the necessary observations, the model would have to summarize success rates over broader clinical disease areas, for example, oncology drugs as opposed to drugs for colorectal cancer.

12.5 Example

In this section we address whether a second confirmatory trial following the positive Phase 3 bevacizumab study in colorectal cancer is necessary. Table 12.8 presents the success rates in Phase 3 clinical trials across a variety of disease areas and the associated ratios of true to false positives. The data come from a report on clinical trial success rates conducted by the Biotechnology Industry Organization (BIO) (Hay et al. 2011). The ratios of true to false positives are computed from the success rates by first making an assumption about the average treatment effect size in the state of nature where the drug is active and then estimating the probability that the drug is active after a successful Phase 2 trial. Specifically, the Phase 3 clinical trial success rate can be expressed as

$$\text{Phase 3 Success Prob.} = p \cdot \Phi\left(z_{\alpha_3} + \left[z_\beta - z_{\alpha_3}\right] \cdot f_\delta\right) + (1-p) \cdot \alpha_3 \quad (12.16)$$

TABLE 12.8

Phase 3 Success Probabilities for a Variety of Clinical Areas along with Calculated Ratios of True to False Positives

	Phase 3 Success Probability	$f_\delta = 0.9$			$f_\delta = 1.0$			$f_\delta = 1.1$		
		Power	p	True+/False+	Power	p	True+/False+	Power	p	True+/False+
Oncology	0.34	0.713	0.531	32	0.8	0.471	28	0.869	0.432	26
CV	0.46	0.713	0.705	68	0.8	0.626	54	0.869	0.575	47
Autoimmune	0.63	0.713	0.952	570	0.8	0.845	175	0.869	0.776	120
Endocrine	0.60	0.713	0.909	284	0.8	0.806	133	0.869	0.741	99
Infectious disease	0.55	0.713	0.836	145	0.8	0.742	92	0.869	0.681	74
Respiratory	0.61	0.713	0.923	343	0.8	0.819	145	0.869	0.752	106
Neurology	0.55	0.713	0.836	145	0.8	0.742	92	0.869	0.681	74

where p is the probability that the drug is active after a successful Phase 2 trial. Solving for p yields

$$p = \frac{\text{Phase 3 Success Prob.} - \alpha_3}{\Phi\left(z_{\alpha_3} + \left[z_\beta - z_{\alpha_3}\right] \cdot f_\delta\right) - \alpha_3} \tag{12.17}$$

Once we have an estimate for p, the ratio of true to false positives is then calculated as

$$\frac{True+}{False+} = \frac{p \cdot \Phi\left(z_{\alpha_3} + \left[z_\beta - z_{\alpha_3}\right] \cdot f_\delta\right)}{(1-p) \cdot \alpha_3} \tag{12.18}$$

When $f_\delta = 1$, the ratios of true to false positives range from 28 for oncology drugs to 175 for drugs that treat autoimmune diseases. Table 12.8 also calculates the ratio of true to false positives for f_δ equal to 0.9 and 1.1, values that represent a treatment effect both less than and greater than what would be used to plan the size of a Phase 3 trial. The larger the average treatment effect size, f_δ, the smaller the ratio of true to false positives. This is due to the fact that a larger treatment effect size is associated with a smaller value for p and hence a larger value for false positives.

Table 12.8 gives us an idea of how the true to false positive rates vary among the different disease areas of drug development. However, it does not enable us to calculate a ratio of true to false positives that incorporates the impact of the Phase 2 design and decision making. Table 12.9 is a first step in that direction. Using the success probabilities in Phase 2 and Phase 3 we can estimate p along with α_2 as follows. First, we can express the Phase 2 and Phase 3 success probabilities as

$$\text{Phase 2 success Prob.} = p \cdot \Phi\left(z_{\alpha_2} + \left[z_\beta - z_{\alpha_3}\right] \cdot f_\delta \cdot \sqrt{f_N}\right) + (1-p) \cdot \alpha_2 \tag{12.19}$$

Phase 3 success Prob.

$$= \frac{p \cdot \Phi\left(z_{\alpha_2} + \left[z_\beta - z_{\alpha_3}\right] \cdot f_\delta \cdot \sqrt{f_N}\right) \cdot \Phi\left(z_{\alpha_3} + \left[z_\beta - z_{\alpha_3}\right] \cdot f_\delta\right) + (1-p) \cdot \alpha_2 \cdot \alpha_3}{p \cdot \Phi\left(z_{\alpha_2} + \left[z_\beta - z_{\alpha_3}\right] \cdot f_\delta \cdot \sqrt{f_N}\right) + (1-p) \cdot \alpha_2} \tag{12.20}$$

Given a value for f_N, the average sample size in Phase 2, there are two unknowns in these two equations: p, the probability of an effective drug entering testing in Phase 2, and α_2, the average critical value for Phase 2

TABLE 12.9

Phase 2 and Phase 3 Success Probabilities for a Variety of Clinical Areas along with Calculated p, α_2, and True to False Positive Rates

	Phase 2 Success Probability	Phase 3 Success Probability	Simple Success Probability	$f_\delta = 1.0$					
				$f_N = 0.10$			$f_N = 0.20$		
				α_2	p	True+/False+	α_2	p	True+/False+
Oncology	0.29	0.34	0.0986	0.220	0.216	22	0.209	0.176	22
CV	0.28	0.46	0.1288	0.181	0.321	41	0.165	0.257	41
Autoimmune	0.30	0.63	0.1890	0.144	0.544	114	0.118	0.444	114
Endocrine	0.36	0.60	0.2160	0.195	0.523	92	0.165	0.438	92
Infectious disease	0.41	0.55	0.2255	0.252	0.474	67	0.222	0.404	67
Respiratory	0.24	0.61	0.1464	0.114	0.484	99	0.095	0.380	98
Neurology	0.32	0.55	0.1760	0.184	0.439	67	0.161	0.359	67

testing. These equations for the Phase 2 and Phase 3 success probabilities can be solved for p and α_2 using numerical techniques. The results are presented in Table 12.9 along with the ratio of true to false positives, which is calculated as

$$
\frac{True+}{False+} = \frac{p \cdot \Phi\left(z_{\alpha_2} - [z_{0.025} - z_{0.80}] \cdot \sqrt{f_N}\right) \cdot \Phi\left(z_{\alpha_3} - [z_{0.025} - z_{0.80}]\right)}{(1-p) \cdot \alpha_2 \cdot \alpha_3} \tag{12.21}
$$

The estimates of p show that molecules in the oncology disease area have the lowest probability of success at the beginning of Phase 2, whereas the estimates of α_2 show that the results from Phase 2 trials are not used as much in oncology as in other clinical areas to screen for molecules that will be taken to Phase 3, the sole exception being the infectious disease area.

Note that when interpreting α_2 it must be kept in mind that this model is unable to separate the increase in probability of a successful Phase 3 that is due to the scientific interpretation of the data collected in Phase 2 and the increase in probability that is simply due to using Phase 2 as a screening trial.

Regardless of how we evaluate the data from the BIO report on clinical trial success rates, the ratio of true to false positives in oncology is lower than in the other major clinical areas. So, we can draw the conclusion that it is less certain that an approval in oncology based on a single Phase 3 trial will provide an effective molecule to patients than it is in the other major disease areas of drug development. For this reason, it may be necessary to require a second Phase 3 trial in the area of oncology in general. Given that the success rate for colorectal cancer as reported by BIO is lower than the success rates for most other cancers, we could more strongly assert the need for a second confirmatory trial in this area.

Now let's focus on the bevacizumab Phase 3 trial in colorectal cancer in particular and assess whether a second Phase 3 confirmatory trial is necessary. Table 12.10 computes the ratio of true to false positives for a bevacizumab approval in colorectal cancer assuming that $p = 0.216$ or 0.176, which are the estimated values for p from the BIO data. The values for α_2 and α_3 are also allowed to vary in the calculation of the ratio of true to false positives.

If we use values for α_2 and α_3 that are typical for Phase 2 and Phase 3 trials, that is, α_2 equals 0.10 and α_3 equals 0.025, then we see that the ratio of power to type 1 error is 24.1 or 31.1 depending on the estimate of p that we chose to use. On the other hand, if we take account of the strong results in Phase 2 as well as Phase 3 and use α_2 equals 0.0685 (the one-sided p-value for survival from the Phase 2 study) and α_3 equals 0.001 (a p-value that is still greater than what was reported for survival in the Phase 3 study), then we see that the ratio of true to false positives is 291 or 375, again depending on

TABLE 12.10

Ratio of True to False Positives for Bevacizumab
Phase 2/3 Program in Colorectal Cancer

f_N	p	α_2	α_3	True+/False+
0.1038961	0.216	0.2000	0.025	23.1
			0.010	49.3
			0.001	279.2
		0.1000	0.025	31.1
			0.010	66.3
			0.001	375.3
		0.0685	0.025	36.0
			0.010	76.8
			0.001	434.6
	0.176	0.2000	0.025	17.9
			0.010	38.2
			0.001	216.4
		0.1000	0.025	24.1
			0.010	51.4
			0.001	291.0
		0.0685	0.025	27.9
			0.010	59.5
			0.001	336.9

the estimate of p. Either of these estimates for the ratio of true to false positives are larger than what we estimated for any clinical area in Table 12.8 and Table 12.9. So, while the general approach to approving drugs leads to a low ratio of true to false positives for oncology as a whole and for colorectal cancer in particular, the results for the bevacizumab Phase 2 and Phase 3 program are sufficiently strong to warrant approval without a second Phase 3 confirmatory trial.

One criticism of the aforementioned approach to estimating the proportion of molecules that ultimately could provide a clinical benefit is that the model assumed all the Phase 2 trials had a control arm for comparison with the experimental treatment. Although this is a reasonable assumption for many clinical areas, in the oncology arena it is not a good assumption to make where many Phase 2 trials have only a single arm. However, even in these single-arm Phase 2 trials, there is almost always an implicit comparison being made with a historical control group. Thus, the probabilities from our model for comparing one group with another are still relevant for the estimation of p.

The results for p and α_2 presented so far rely on the reported success rates for Phase 2 and Phase 3 trials. In this chapter we pointed out what we could determine using maximum likelihood if for each molecule we had summary Z-statistics for both Phase 2 and Phase 3 when the studies are undertaken.

If we had this data and applied the model described in Equation, (12.15), then we could estimate the impact of a Phase 2 trial used as a screen for Phase 3 on the probability of a successful Phase 3 trial as well as the additional increase that was due to the scientific interpretation of the Phase 2 results. This sort of data could be collected by regulatory agencies as part of their requirements for companies studying new molecular entities in humans and would facilitate the evaluation of clinical trial evidence provided by drug companies to support marketing approval.

References

Chan, J.K., Ueda, S.M., Suglyama, V.E., et al. 2008. Analysis of phase II studies on targeted agents and subsequent phase III trials: What are the predictors for success? *J Clin Oncol* 26(9):1511–1518.

DiMasi, J.A., Feldman, L., Seckler, A., Wilson, A. 2010. Trends in risks associated with new drug development: Success rates for investigational drugs. *Nature, Clin Pharmacol Ther* 87(3):272–277.

Hay, M., Rosenthal, J., Thomas, D., Craighead, J. 2011. BIO/BioMedTracker clinical trials success rate study. http://insidebioia.files.wordpress.com/2011/02/bio-ceo-biomedtracker-bio-study-handout-final-2-15-2011.pdf.

Section III

Additional Topics

13

Maximize Efficiency Subject to a Constraint on the Ratio of True to False Positives

It is interesting to think about the impact on the drug development process if drug companies and regulators both know that marketing approval cannot be attained unless it has been shown that the ratio of true to false positives exceeds a prespecified level. The first thing to note in this regard is that maximizing the ratio of true to false positives is not the same as maximizing efficiency. Figure 13.1 compares the efficiency and ratio of true to false positives for various Phase 2 designs when the total sample size in Phase 2 and Phase 3 is held fixed.

For Phase 2 studies with a high α-value there is not much difference between the size of the Phase 2 study that maximizes efficiency and the size that maximizes the ratio of true to false positives. On the other hand, for Phase 2 studies with a low α-value, for example, 0.05, there can be a big difference, in this case 0.30 versus 0.45, in the fraction of the total sample size in Phase 2 that maximizes the efficiency and the ratio of true to false positives.

Now let's examine how a drug company would behave if it attempts to maximize efficiency subject to the constraint that the ratio of true to false positives equals the level K. That is, the drug company maximizes

$$\text{Efficiency} = \frac{p \cdot \Phi\left(z_{\alpha_2} - \left(z_{\alpha_3} - z_\beta\right) \cdot f_\delta \cdot \sqrt{f_{N_2}}\right) \cdot \Phi\left(z_{\alpha_3^*} - \left(z_{\alpha_3} - z_\beta\right) \cdot f_\delta \cdot \sqrt{f_{N_3}}\right)}{N\left(f_{N_2} + f_{N_3} \cdot \left[p \cdot \Phi\left(z_{\alpha_2} - \left(z_{\alpha_3} - z_\beta\right) \cdot f_\delta \cdot \sqrt{f_{N_2}}\right) + (1-p) \cdot \alpha_2\right]\right)} \quad (13.1)$$

subject to the following constraint:

$$T+/F+ = \frac{p \cdot \Phi\left(z_{\alpha_2} - \left(z_{\alpha_3} - z_\beta\right) \cdot f_\delta \cdot \sqrt{f_{N_2}}\right) \cdot \Phi\left(z_{\alpha_3^*} - \left(z_{\alpha_3} - z_\beta\right) \cdot f_\delta \cdot \sqrt{f_{N_3}}\right)}{(1-p) \cdot \alpha_2 \cdot \alpha_3^*} = K \quad (13.2)$$

Using the constraint we can solve for α_3^*

$$\alpha_3^* = \frac{p \cdot \Phi\left(z_{\alpha_2} - \left(z_{\alpha_3} - z_\beta\right) \cdot f_\delta \cdot \sqrt{f_{N_2}}\right) \cdot \Phi\left(z_{\alpha_3^*} - \left(z_{\alpha_3} - z_\beta\right) \cdot f_\delta \cdot \sqrt{f_{N_3}}\right)}{(1-p) \cdot \alpha_2 \cdot K} \quad (13.3)$$

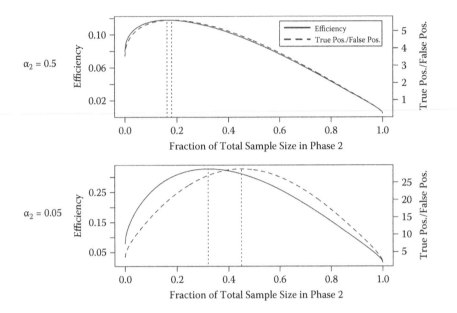

FIGURE 13.1
Efficiency and the ratio of true to false positives as a function of the fraction of the total sample size used in Phase 2 and Phase 3.

and if we assume that the Phase 3 study is powered at 80 percent, then α_3^* equals

$$\alpha_3^* = \frac{p \cdot \Phi\left(z_{\alpha_2} - \left(z_{\alpha_3} - z_\beta\right) \cdot f_\delta \cdot \sqrt{f_{N_2}}\right) \cdot 0.80}{(1-p) \cdot \alpha_2 \cdot K} \tag{13.4}$$

Now we can go ahead and further solve for f_{N_3} from the equation

$$\Phi\left(z_{\alpha_3^*} - \left(z_{\alpha_3} - z_\beta\right) \cdot f_\delta \cdot \sqrt{f_{N_3}}\right) = 0.80 \tag{13.5}$$

which yields

$$f_{N_3} = \left(\frac{z_{\alpha_3^*} - \Phi^{-1}(0.80)}{\left(z_{\alpha_3} - z_\beta\right) \cdot f_\delta}\right)^2 \tag{13.6}$$

Using the relations derived earlier from the constraint on the ratio of true to false positives described in Equation (13.2), Figure 13.2 presents efficiency as a function of the Phase 2 design. Here, the probability that the drug is indeed effective is taken to be 0.10.

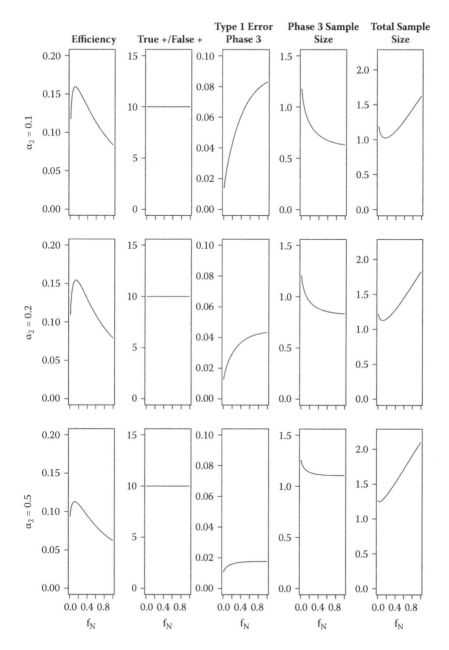

FIGURE 13.2
Efficiency as a function of f_N in Phase 2 when the ratio of true positives to false positives is held constant.

What is interesting to note in this figure is how the value for f_N that maximizes efficiency is relatively stable at around 0.15, while the type 1 error in Phase 2 ranges from 0.10 to 0.50. That is, the Phase 2 trial should be conducted with approximately 15 percent of the Phase 3 sample size regardless of the level of testing in Phase 2. Further, the type 1 error that maximizes the efficiency among those levels included in Figure 13.2 is 0.10. This will maximize the efficiency after accounting for the requirement from regulators that the combined Phase 2/Phase 3 program achieve a specific level, in this case 10, for the ratio of true to false positives.

14

Power of the Log Rank Test to Detect Improvement in Mean Survival Time and the Impact of Censoring

A commonly used procedure for comparing two survival distributions is the log rank test. One reason that the log rank test is often used is that it can handle censored observations. That is, it can account for subjects who have been randomized and treated but for whom the event of interest has not occurred at the time of the analysis. Doksum (1969), Janssen (1999), and Schoenfeld (1981) have investigated the power of the log rank test. The ability to handle censored observations also introduces a difficulty when interpreting the results of the log rank test. Oftentimes, the events of interest do not come from the whole range of the survival distribution but instead only arise from those subjects who are the first to have an event. We are therefore forced to assume that the experience for the subjects who had an event early can be extrapolated to the experience for subjects who will have an event late to draw conclusions related to how the two survival distributions as a whole compare.

Unfortunately, the treatment benefit that is observed early does not always match the treatment benefit that comes later. The experience from the NSABP C-08 study reported by Allegra (2010), provides an example of how the treatment effect can change over time. Over the first 15 months of the study, the hazard ratio was 0.66 ($p < 0.0001$) and post 15 months the hazard ratio was 1.2 ($p = 0.07$). This treatment by time interaction was statistically significant at the $p < 0.0001$ level.

To aid the interpretation of the log rank test with regard to the survival time of all subjects treated, this chapter determines the minimum power of the log rank test for a given difference in the mean survival time between the treatment and control arms with particular attention paid to the impact of censoring. These results will help regulators gauge how much risk they are assuming with an approval based on the log rank test with censored observations by determining the minimum power that may be attained among pairs of survival curves with the given difference in mean survival time that is of interest. If this minimum power is too low, then the evidence in favor of the treatment improving survival may not be sufficient, just as a statistically significant yet underpowered comparison using the difference in means may not be sufficient to gain marketing approval.

14.1 Setup

To determine the minimum power that can be attained by the log rank test for a given difference in mean survival times we would ideally seek to minimize the expected value of the log rank test among the family of all treatment and control distributions where the mean survival time in the control arm is $1/\lambda_C$ and the mean survival time in the treatment arm is $1/\lambda_T$. By finding the minimum expected value of the log rank test among this family of pairs of distributions we could then determine the minimum power associated with a given level of the treatment effect. Unfortunately, the minimization of the log rank test over this family of pairs of distributions is not very informative since the pairs of distributions that achieve the minimum value of the log rank test are those with almost all of the probability density for the treatment distribution at 0 and the remaining amount of probability at a survival time that would make the overall mean equal to $1/\lambda_T$. So, instead of minimizing the log rank test over this family of treatment and control distributions we reduce the family of distributions by setting the treatment distribution to be some arbitrary distribution, for example, the exponential distribution with mean $1/\lambda_T$ or a targeted survival curve based on the anticipated control distribution and the minimum clinically meaningful treatment effect, λ_T/λ_C. The family of control distributions is then set to be all survival distributions with mean $1/\lambda_C$. Within this family of control distributions we identify the distribution that minimizes the log rank test. The minimum power of the log rank test is then determined by calculating the power relative to this member of the control family. In essence, we are asking how close can the control distribution be to the specified arbitrary treatment distribution measured by how low the power is and still be consistent with a mean survival time of $1/\lambda_C$.

We will show that when the treatment distribution is exponential and there is no censoring, the control distribution that minimizes the log rank statistic is approximately an exponential distribution and hence the proportional hazards assumption is satisfied. In this regard, it is interesting to recall as outlined in Appendix D that the log rank test maximizes the power among all rank-based procedures under proportional hazards. When there is considerable censoring prior to the median survival time of the treatment and control arms, then the control distribution that minimizes the log rank statistic can be very different from an exponential distribution with hazard λ_C. Thus, if the study was powered under the proportional hazards assumption, there is considerable risk to the regulator that the study is underpowered for clinically meaningful treatment effects on the mean survival time scale. On the other hand, when the censoring encompasses most of the range of the survival distribution, the control distribution that minimizes the log rank statistic once again approximates the exponential distribution and thus if the study was powered under the proportional hazards assumption, there is little risk the study will be underpowered to detect the specified difference in mean survival time between the treatment and control arms. Thus, a regulator should pay close attention to the pattern of censoring in relation to the survival distribution when assessing how much risk is assumed in terms of the improvement in mean survival time when a new molecule is approved based on the log rank test.

14.2 Minimizing the Log Rank Test

Using the notation of Fleming and Harrington (1991), the expected value of the log rank statistic can be expressed as

$$LR = \int_0^\infty E\left\{K(s)\cdot\left(\frac{f_1(s)}{1-F_1(s)} - \frac{f_2(s)}{1-F_2(s)}\right)\right\}\cdot ds \tag{14.1}$$

where $f_i(s)$ and $F_i(s)$ represent, respectively, the density and cumulative distribution function for the survival times in group i and $K(s) = \dfrac{\bar{Y}_1(s)\cdot\bar{Y}_2(s)}{\bar{Y}_1(s)+\bar{Y}_2(s)}$. Note that $\bar{Y}_i(s)$ represents the number of subjects at risk in group i at time s. Assuming no censoring, we can rewrite the log rank test as

$$LR = \int_0^\infty E\left\{\frac{\bar{Y}_1(s)\cdot\bar{Y}_2(s)}{\bar{Y}_1(s)+\bar{Y}_2(s)}\cdot\left(\frac{f_1(s)}{[1-F_1(s)]} - \frac{f_2(s)}{[1-F_2(s)]}\right)\right\}\cdot ds \tag{14.2}$$

$$= \int_0^\infty E[1+r(s)]\cdot\frac{n_1(1-F_1(s))\cdot n_2(1-F_2(s))}{n_1(1-F_1(s))+n_2(1-F_2(s))}\cdot\left(\frac{f_1(s)}{[1-F_1(s)]} - \frac{f_2(s)}{[1-F_2(s)]}\right)\cdot ds \tag{14.3}$$

$$= \int_0^\infty E[1+r(s)]\cdot\left(\frac{n_1\cdot n_2\cdot(1-F_2(s))\cdot f_1(s)}{n_1(1-F_1(s))+n_2(1-F_2(s))} - \frac{n_1\cdot n_2\cdot(1-F_1(s))\cdot f_2(s)}{n_1(1-F_1(s))+n_2(1-F_2(s))}\right)\cdot ds \tag{14.4}$$

where $\max_{0<s<T} r(s) = o_p(1)$ for any T with $F_1(T) > 0$ and $F_2(T) > 0$, see Appendix E. Since $r(s)$ is also bounded over the interval $[0,T]$, $E[\max_{0<s<T} r(s)] \to 0$ as n_1 and $n_2 \to \infty$.

To minimize the log rank test among all control distributions with the same expected survival time, Lagrange multipliers can be used to form the following objective function:

$$\int_0^\infty E[1+r(s)]\cdot\left[\frac{n_1\cdot n_2\cdot(1-F_2(s))\cdot f_1(s)}{n_1(1-F_1(s))+n_2(1-F_2(s))}-\frac{n_1\cdot n_2\cdot(1-F_1(s))\cdot f_2(s)}{n_1(1-F_1(s))+n_2(1-F_2(s))}\cdot ds\right]$$

$$-\eta\left[\int_0^\infty(1-F_2(s))\cdot ds-C\right]$$

$$\text{(14.5)}$$

We will treat this objective function as infinitely parameterized by $F_2(s)$ and the first partial derivatives of this objective function with respect to $F_2(s)$ will be used to find the distribution that minimizes the log rank test as in Cover and Thomas (1991). Note that the derivative of $f_2(s)$ with respect to $F_2(s)$ cannot be determined. So strictly speaking, we cannot find the distribution that minimizes the log rank test using this approach. However, if we change the problem and treat $f_2(s)$ as fixed then we can get a solution that may be close to the distribution that minimizes the log rank test since there is only a small difference in the objective functions. Doing so yields

$$\frac{E[1+r(s)]\cdot n_1\cdot n_2\cdot\left[-n_1 f_1(s)-n_2 f_2(s)\right]\cdot\left[1-F_1(s)\right]}{\left[n_1(1-F_1(s))+n_2(1-F_2(s))\right]^2}+\eta=0 \qquad\text{(14.6)}$$

$$\frac{E[1+r(s)]\cdot\left[n_1 f_1(s)+n_2 f_2(s)\right]}{\left[n_1(1-F_1(s))+n_2(1-F_2(s))\right]^2}=\frac{\eta/(n_1 n_2)}{\left[1-F_1(s)\right]} \qquad\text{(14.7)}$$

which can be expressed as

$$\frac{\partial}{\partial s}\left[n_1(1-F_1(s))+n_2(1-F_2(s))\right]^{-1}=\frac{\eta/(n_1 n_2)}{E[1+r(s)]\cdot\left[1-F_1(s)\right]} \qquad\text{(14.8)}$$

which implies that

$$n_1(1-F_1(s))+n_2(1-F_2(s))=\cfrac{1}{\displaystyle\int\frac{\eta/(n_1 n_2)}{E[1+r(s)]\cdot\left[1-F_1(s)\right]}\cdot ds+D} \qquad\text{(14.9)}$$

With $F_1(s)=1-e^{-\lambda_1 x}$, it can be concluded that

$$n_1(1-F_1(s))+n_2(1-F_2(s))=\cfrac{1}{\displaystyle\int\frac{\eta/(n_1 n_2)}{E[1+r(s)]\cdot\exp(-\lambda_1\cdot s)}\cdot ds+D} \qquad\text{(14.10)}$$

$$\rightarrow\cfrac{1}{\cfrac{\eta/\lambda_1}{n_1 n_2}\exp(\lambda_1\cdot s)+D} \qquad\text{(14.11)}$$

since $E\left[\max_{0<s<T} r(s)\right] \to 0$ as n_1 and $n_2 \to \infty$. Note that setting $s = 0$ results in $D = \dfrac{1}{n_1 + n_2} - \dfrac{\eta / \lambda_1}{n_1 n_2}$. Further, Equation (14.11) can be solved for $1 - F_2(s)$ to obtain

$$1 - F_2(s) = \frac{1}{\dfrac{\eta / \lambda_1}{n_1} \cdot \exp(\lambda_1 \cdot s) + \dfrac{n_2}{n_1 + n_2} - \dfrac{\eta / \lambda_1}{n_1}} - \frac{n_1 / n_2}{\exp(\lambda_1 \cdot s)} \qquad (14.12)$$

Now the value of $\eta / n_1 \lambda_1$ can be determined from the constraint

$$\int_0^\infty (1 - F_2(s)) \cdot ds = C = \frac{1}{\lambda_2} \qquad (14.13)$$

$$\int_0^\infty 1 - F_2(s) \cdot ds = \int_0^\infty \left[\frac{1}{\dfrac{\eta / \lambda_1}{n_1} \cdot \exp(\lambda_1 \cdot s) + \dfrac{n_2}{n_1 + n_2} - \dfrac{\eta / \lambda_1}{n_1}} - \frac{n_1 / n_2}{\exp(\lambda_1 \cdot s)} \right] \cdot ds \qquad (14.14)$$

$$= \int_0^\infty \frac{1}{\dfrac{\eta / \lambda_1}{n_1} \cdot \exp(\lambda_1 \cdot s) + \dfrac{n_2}{n_1 + n_2} - \dfrac{\eta / \lambda_1}{n_1}} ds - \frac{n_1 / n_2}{\lambda_1} \qquad (14.15)$$

Substituting $u = \exp(\lambda_1 \cdot s)$ leads to

$$= \int_1^\infty \frac{1}{\dfrac{\eta / \lambda_1}{n_1} \cdot u + \dfrac{n_2}{n_1 + n_2} - \dfrac{\eta / \lambda_1}{n_1}} \frac{du}{\lambda u} - \frac{n_1 / n_2}{\lambda_1} \qquad (14.16)$$

$$= \int_1^\infty \frac{du}{\left(\dfrac{\eta}{n_1} \cdot u + \dfrac{n_2 \lambda}{n_1 + n_2} - \dfrac{\eta}{n_1} \right) u} - \frac{n_1 / n_2}{\lambda_1} \qquad (14.17)$$

Integrating by parts results in

$$\log\left(\frac{n_1 n_2}{n_1 + n_2} \frac{\lambda_1}{\eta} \right) \frac{n_1}{\dfrac{n_1 n_2}{n_1 + n_2} \lambda_1 - \eta} - \frac{n_1 / n_2}{\lambda_1} \qquad (14.18)$$

Thus

$$\log \frac{\dfrac{n_1 n_2}{n_1 + n_2} \dfrac{\lambda_1}{\eta}}{\left(\dfrac{n_1 n_2}{n_1 + n_2} \lambda_1 - \eta \right)} - \frac{n_1 / n_2}{\lambda_1} = \frac{1}{\lambda_2} \qquad (14.19)$$

and Equation (14.20) can be used to solve numerically for $\eta/(n_1\lambda_1)$ and thus determine the control distribution that minimizes the log rank test

$$\frac{\lambda_1}{\lambda_2} + \frac{n_1}{n_2} = \log\left(\frac{n_1+n_2}{n_2}\frac{\eta}{n_1\lambda_1}\right)\frac{1}{\dfrac{\eta}{n_1\lambda_1} - \dfrac{n_2}{n_1+n_2}} \qquad (14.20)$$

Note that if $\lambda_2 \to \lambda_1$, then $1 - F_2(s) \to \exp(-\lambda_1 \cdot s)$. This follows from the fact that $\dfrac{\eta}{n_1\lambda_1} \to \dfrac{n_2}{n_1+n_2}$ since

$$\lim_{\frac{\eta}{n_1\lambda_1} \to \frac{n_2}{n_1+n_2}} \log\left(\frac{n_1+n_2}{n_2}\frac{\eta}{n_1\lambda_1}\right)\frac{1}{\dfrac{\eta}{n_1\lambda_1} - \dfrac{n_2}{n_1+n_2}}$$

$$= \lim_{\frac{\eta}{n_1\lambda_1} \to \frac{n_2}{n_1+n_2}} \frac{1/\left(\dfrac{\eta}{n_1\lambda_1}\right)}{1} = \frac{n_1+n_2}{n_2} \qquad (14.21)$$

Consequently, as $\lambda_2 \to \lambda_1$

$$1 - F_2(s) \to \frac{1}{\dfrac{n_2}{n_1+n_2}\exp(\lambda_1 \cdot s) + \dfrac{n_2}{n_1+n_2} - \dfrac{n_2}{n_1+n_2}} - \frac{n_1/n_2}{\exp(\lambda_1 \cdot s)} = \exp(-\lambda_1 \cdot s)$$

$$\qquad (14.22)$$

14.3 Examples

Figure 14.1 is a graph of the control distribution that minimizes the log rank test determined according to (14.20) along with the treatment distribution and the censoring distribution. Table 14.1 presents the power of the log rank test under the distribution for the control arm that minimizes the expected value of the log rank test along with several other distributions to assess whether the power of the log rank test is indeed minimized at the identified distribution. In addition to the power, Table 14.1 presents the proportion of subjects in the control arm that had an event and the expected value of the control arm. The powers for these various distributions are computed by simulation. The hazard is assumed to be 0.15 (median time = 4.6, mean time = 6.67) in the treatment arm and 0.30 (median time 2.3, mean time = 3.33) in the control arm for a hazard ratio of 0.5. It is assumed that there are 36 subjects per arm and 3000 replications were undertaken to estimate the power. Note that the power

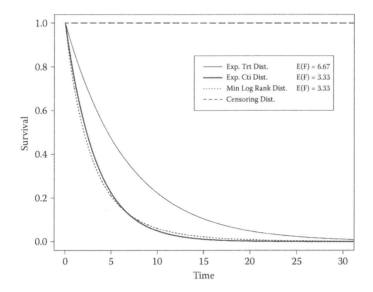

FIGURE 14.1
Control distribution that minimizes the power of the log rank test, no censoring.

TABLE 14.1

Power of the Log Rank Test for Various Control Distributions with the Same Mean Survival, No Censoring

Distribution	Power	Proportion with Event	Expected Value
Calculated	0.773	1.000	3.332
exp(x,.333)[a]	0.818	1.000	3.338
Gamma(60,18)[b]	0.988	1.000	3.338
Gamma(12,3.6)	0.982	1.000	3.338
Gamma(3,.9)	0.963	1.000	3.338
Gamma(1,.3)	0.900	1.000	3.338
exp(1.33 + x,.5)	0.952	1.000	3.338
exp(2.83 + x,0.5)	0.987	1.000	3.338
Normal(3,0.5)[c]	0.965	1.000	3.338
Normal(3,0.1)	0.972	1.000	3.338

[a] exp(x, rate).
[b] Gamma(shape, rate).
[c] Normal(mean, SD).

under the distribution for the control arm that we calculated would minimize the log rank statistic is very close to the power under the exponential alternative in the family as we anticipated. Further, the power for the other distributions we used for the control are greater than the power for the distribution we determined would minimize the log rank statistic.

14.4 Censoring

We can usually anticipate what the censoring distribution for a study will look like from the planned enrollment rates and the duration of the follow-up period. Here, the impact of the duration of follow-up on the minimum value of the log rank test is explored.

We can modify the equations presented earlier to account for censoring as follows:

$$LR = \int_0^\infty \left[1 + r(s)\right] \cdot \left(\begin{array}{c} \dfrac{n_1 n_2 \left[1 - F_2(s)\right] \cdot \left[1 - G(s)\right]}{n_1 \left[1 - F_1(s)\right] + n_2 \left[1 - F_2(s)\right]} \cdot f_1(s) \\[3mm] - \dfrac{n_1 n_2 \left[1 - F_1(s)\right] \cdot \left[1 - G(s)\right]}{n_1 \left[1 - F_1(s)\right] + n_2 \left[1 - F_2(s)\right]} \cdot f_2(s) \end{array} \right) \cdot ds \quad (14.23)$$

$$\frac{\partial}{\partial s} \left(n_1 \cdot \left[1 - F_1(s)\right] + n_2 \cdot \left[1 - F_2(s)\right] \right)^{-1} = \frac{\eta / (n_1 n_2)}{\left[1 + r(s)\right] \cdot \left[1 - F_1(s)\right] \cdot \left[1 - G(s)\right]} \quad (14.24)$$

$$1 - F_2(s) = \frac{1}{\dfrac{\eta}{n_1} \displaystyle\int_0^s \exp(\lambda_1 \cdot x) / \left[1 - G(x)\right] \cdot dx + \dfrac{n_2}{n_1 + n_2}} - \frac{n_1 / n_2}{\exp(\lambda_1 \cdot s)} \quad (14.25)$$

Here, η is determined so that the expected value of $F_2 = 1/\lambda_2$.

Figure 14.2 describes the distribution that is proposed to minimize the log rank test when there is censoring over the range of the survival distribution, and Table 14.2 calculates the power of the log rank test under this distribution along with several others. The actual hazards for the treatment and control distributions are the same as for the example in Figure 14.1, 0.15 and 0.30, respectively. There are 40 subjects per arm and 3000 replications were undertaken to estimate the power. Note that there is very little difference between the distribution we calculated would minimize the log rank test and the corresponding exponential distribution. Further, note in Table 14.2 that the power of the log rank test is minimized with the exponential distribution and with the distribution we calculated would minimize the log rank test. Thus, when censoring spans the range of survival times as in this example, the power to detect a difference between a treatment and control distribution consistent with the given difference in mean survival will be at least as great as what is calculated from the log rank test under the proportional hazards assumption.

In the final example presented in Figure 14.3 and Table 14.3, there is considerable censoring taking place prior to the median of the control arm. The control and treatment arms have hazards of 0.15 and 0.30 as before,

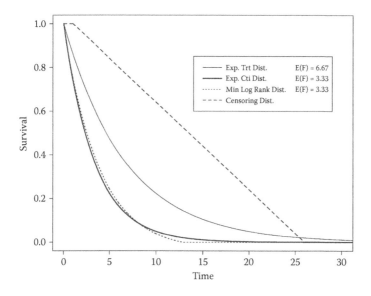

FIGURE 14.2
Control distribution that minimizes the power of the log rank test, censoring over the range of survival times.

TABLE 14.2

Power of the Log Rank Test for Various Control Distributions with the Same Mean Survival; Censoring over the Range of Survival Times

Distribution	Power	Proportion with Event	Expected Value
Calculated	0.803	0.901	3.333
exp(x,.333)[a]	0.804	0.901	3.338
Gamma(60,18)[b]	0.979	0.906	3.338
Gamma(12,3.6)	0.969	0.906	3.338
Gamma(3,.9)	0.939	0.906	3.338
Gamma(1,.3)	0.906	0.901	3.338
exp(1.33 + x,.5)	0.930	0.906	3.338
exp(2.83 + x,0.5)	0.977	0.906	3.338
Normal(3,0.5)[c]	0.937	0.906	3.338
Normal(3,0.1)	0.949	0.906	3.338

[a] exp(x, rate).
[b] Gamma(shape, rate).
[c] Normal(mean, SD).

the number of subjects per arm is 67, and the number of replications under-taken in the simulation to estimate the power is 3000. Note the substantial reduction in power for the distribution calculated to minimize the power of the log rank test in comparison to the exponential control distribution with the same mean. The reduction in power is due to most of the events

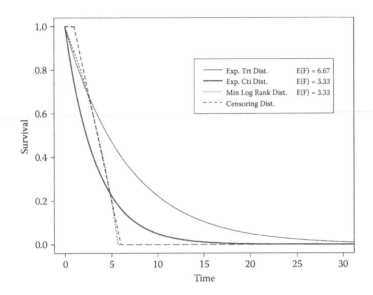

FIGURE 14.3
Control distribution that minimizes the power of the log rank test, considerable censoring prior to the median.

TABLE 14.3

Power of the Log Rank Test for Various Control Distributions with the Same Mean Survival; Considerable Censoring Prior to the Median

Distribution	Power	Proportion with Event	Expected Value
Calculated	0.287	0.519	3.331
exp(x,.333)[a]	0.811	0.616	3.338
Gamma(60,18)[b]	0.818	0.532	3.338
Gamma(12,3.6)	0.727	0.533	3.338
Gamma(3,.9)	0.736	0.557	3.338
Gamma(1,.3)	0.904	0.616	3.338
exp(1.33 + x,.5)	0.812	0.571	3.338
exp(2.83 + x,0.5)	0.797	0.533	3.338
Normal(3,0.5)[c]	0.467	0.532	3.338
Normal(3,0.1)	0.586	0.532	3.338

[a] exp(x, rate).
[b] Gamma(shape, rate).
[c] Normal(mean, SD).

occurring where censoring is taking place, that is, when less weight is given to the event by the log rank test. Thus in this situation, if the power for the log rank test is calculated based on the proportional hazards assumption, there can be treatment and control distributions with the given difference in mean survival times for which the power of the log rank test is much lower than per the proportional hazards assumption. Thus, the regulator faces the risk that the strength of evidence in favor of the drug in a positive study is not as great as the power calculation suggests, since there are clinically meaningful alternatives that are underpowered.

14.5 Survival Benefit in the Bevacizumab Phase 3 Colorectal Cancer Trial

The bevacizumab Phase 3 clinical trial in colorectal cancer was introduced in Chapter 1. The study was designed to detect an improvement in the median overall survival time from 15 months to 20 months, which corresponds to a hazard ratio of 0.75 under an exponential model. Three hundred eighty-five deaths were deemed necessary to have 80 percent power to detect this treatment effect with a one-sided type 1 error of 0.025.

To start this analysis, a piecewise exponential function was used to approximate the survival curves reported in Hurwitz et al. (2004). The parameters for the piecewise exponential functions corresponding to the IFL + Placebo and IFL + Bevacizumab arms are presented in Table 14.4.

The approximation out to 24.5 months is based on the Kaplan Meier survival curves reported in Hurwitz et al. (2004). After 24.5 months the data from this study are too weak to support an estimate of survival. Instead, the data reported in Kopetz et al. (2009) for the period 1998 to 2000 was used to estimate the survival past 24.5 months in the IFL + Placebo arm. Survival past 24.5 months in the IFL + Bevacizumab arm was determined by setting the hazard ratio relative to the IFL + Placebo arm at 0.75. This represents the minimal improvement in the hazard ratio that would be considered meaningful. The piecewise exponential survival curves described in Table 14.4 are presented in Figure 14.4.

As presented in Figure 14.4, the expected survival time is 25.7 months in the IFL + Placebo arm and 34.1 months in the IFL + Bevacizumab arm. At the

TABLE 14.4

Piecewise Exponential Approximation to the Bevacizumab Phase 3 Colorectal Trial Kaplan Meier Survival Curves

Time Period	Source	IFL + Placebo	IFL + Bevacizumab
0–5 months	Hurwitz et al. 2004	0.0211	0.0211
5–10 months	Hurwitz et al. 2004	0.0497	0.0236
10–15.6 months	Hurwitz et al. 2004	0.0602	0.0398
15.6–20.3 months	Hurwitz et al. 2004	0.0475	0.0525
20.3–24.5 months	Hurwitz et al. 2004	0.0475	0.0472
> 24.5 months	Kopetz et al. 2009	0.033	0.0248

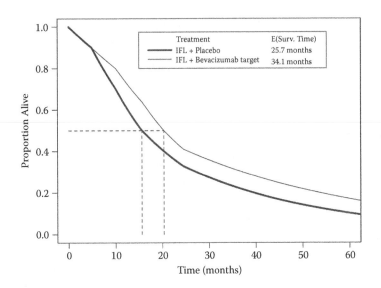

FIGURE 14.4
Piecewise exponential approximation to the bevacizumab Phase 3 colorectal cancer survival curves.

time that the Hurwitz et al. (2004) study was reported no one knew exactly what the survival for IFL + Bevacizumab would be past 25 months since there was heavy censoring starting at that time. So the actual expected survival in this arm is uncertain and *a fortiori* it is not certain that the expected survival in the IFL + Bevacizumab arm is longer than in the control arm. This uncertainty in how the expected survival time compares between the two arms is quantified to some degree in Figure 14.5, which presents the power to detect a survival difference between the reported/assumed IFL + Bevacizumab arm and the worst case control (smallest p-value relative to the log rank test) for a range of expected survival times in the control arm. Note that the power was computed using a sample of 200 simulated studies. In Figure 14.5 it can be seen that there is no power to detect a difference between the worst-case control with a mean survival time of 21 months and the survival curve for the IFL + Bevacizumab arm. So, although the log rank test may be significant at this point there is not adequate power to draw the conclusion that the mean survival time has been increased. This parallels the situation where an underpowered study that reports a significant p-value for the comparison of two treatments is not sufficient evidence for regulatory approval to market the drug. Noting that the log rank test is not powered to detect a difference with the least favorable control is another way of saying that the observed survival curve for the IFL + Bevacizumab arm may be no different than the IFL + Placebo arm in terms of mean survival time. So, with the extent of follow-up reported in Hurwitz et al., (2004)

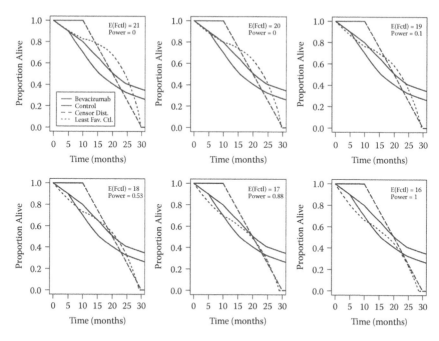

FIGURE 14.5
Control distributions with a range of expected survival times that minimize the log rank test relative to the treatment distribution.

the study is not sufficiently powered to determine whether the expected survival time is greater than 21 months, let alone the 25 months estimated for the control arm.

Figure 14.6 illustrates the impact of additional follow-up on the power of the log rank test. As would be expected, additional follow-up increases the power. When there is 56 months of follow-up on all subjects there is approximately 80 percent power versus the least favorable control. Note that 20 percent of the subjects in the IFL + Bevacizumab arm would be alive at 56 months according to the survival curves in Figure 14.4. At this point, a significant log rank test would enable one to conclude that the drug has prolonged expected survival.

14.6 Discussion

As we have previously noted, one could argue that the decision to grant marketing approval for a new drug should be made when there is adequate power to detect a treatment benefit for all clinically meaningful alternatives

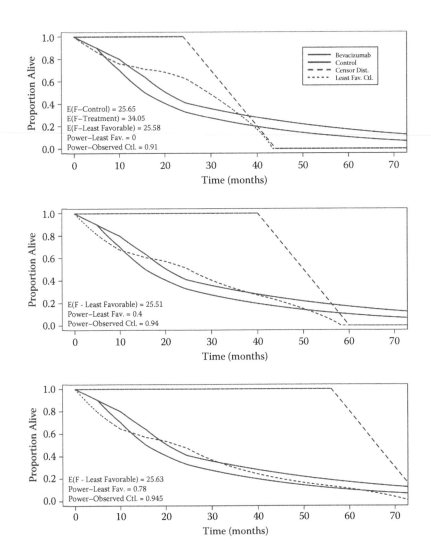

FIGURE 14.6
The impact of additional follow-up on the power of the log rank test versus the least favorable distribution.

under consideration. The regulatory preference for a test based on a simple difference in means over a covariate adjusted assessment of treatment benefit can at least in part be explained by noting that the simple difference in means minimizes the maximum variance relative to a covariate adjusted analyses. We noted earlier that the control distribution that minimizes the log rank test when there is complete follow-up is exponential when the treatment distribution is also exponential. When there is considerable censoring prior to the median of the control arm, the control distribution that minimizes the power of the log rank test among all controls with the same mean survival will be substantially different than the exponential distribution in the family of control distributions and hence the power will be less than what is calculated under proportional hazards. So, one approach for granting marketing approval for a new drug is to require pivotal studies using the log rank test for the primary analysis of a time to event endpoint have adequate follow-up as well as adequate power. Without such extended follow-up, clinically meaningful alternatives will be underpowered and hence the ratio of true positives to false positives may be less than is acceptable for some states of nature where the drug provides benefit to patients.

References

Allegra, C.J., Yothers, G., et al. 2010. Phase III trial assessing bevacizumab in stages II and III carcinoma of the colon. Results of NSABP Protocol C-08. *J Clin Oncol* 29(1):11–16.

Cover, T.M., Thomas, J.A. 1991. *Elements of Information Theory*. New York: Wiley.

Doksum, K. 1969. Minimax results for IFRA scale alternatives. *Ann Math Stat* 40:1778–1783.

Fleming, T.R., Harrington, D.P. 1991. *Counting Processes and Survival Analysis*. New York: Wiley.

Hurwitz, H., Fehrenbacher, L., et al. 2004. Bevacizumab plus irinotecan, fluorouracil, and leucovorin for metastatic colorectal cancer. *N Engl J Med* 350:2335–2342.

Janssen, A. 1999. Testing nonparametric statistical functionals with applications to rank tests. *J Stat Plann Inference* 81:71–93.

Kopetz, S., Chang, G., et al. 2009. Improved survival in metastatic colorectal cancer is associated with adoption of hepatic resection and improved chemotherapy. *J Clin Oncol* 27(22):3677–3683.

Schoenfeld, D. 1981. The asymptotic properties of nonparametric tests for comparing survival distributions. *Biometrika* 68:316–319.

15

Adaptive Phase 2/3 Designs

Adaptive Phase 2/3 studies are clinical trials that are initiated at the point where Phase 1 testing is complete, first answer questions about dose, study population, and so on, and then continue on to provide the definitive evidence of clinical benefit that is required to support drug approval. Bauer (1989) conceived of adaptive trial designs in terms of combining p-values from various stages of the trial in a manner that is defined *a priori*.

The feature of an adaptive Phase 2/3 study that makes it appealing is that it takes fewer subjects in the clinical trial program as a whole to achieve an 80 to 90 percent powered trial, the standard of evidence that is required to obtain marketing approval. In this chapter we evaluate the impact on drug development of allowing evidence from Phase 2 to be used in an adaptive Phase 2/3 design as part of the information that is normally provided by a separate 80 percent powered Phase 3 trial. First, we will evaluate how the drug company's behavior will change by looking at efficiency. Then, we will evaluate the impact on the ratio of true to false positives of allowing evidence from Phase 2 to support approval.

15.1 Impact of Adaptive Designs on Drug Company Behavior

To model a drug company's behavior when faced with the option of an adaptive trial design we will assume that the drug company will attempt to maximize the efficiency expressed as

$$\eta = \frac{p \cdot \Phi\left(z_{\alpha_2} - \left[z_{\alpha_3} - z_\beta\right] \cdot f_\delta \cdot \sqrt{f_N}\right) \cdot \Phi\left(z_{\alpha_3} - \left[z_{\alpha_3} - z_\beta\right] \cdot f_\delta \cdot \sqrt{f_{N_{Adapt}}}\right)}{C + N \cdot \left[f_N + f_{N_{Adapt}} \cdot \left\{p \cdot \Phi\left(z_{\alpha_2} - \left[z_{\alpha_3} - z_\beta\right] \cdot f_\delta \cdot \sqrt{f_N}\right) + (1-p) \cdot \alpha_2\right\}\right]} \quad (15.1)$$

where $f_{N_{Adapt}}$ represents the fraction of the normal Phase 3 sample size that needs to be enrolled to complete Phase 3 testing using an adaptive design. Since this is an adaptive Phase 2/3 design, we will treat the first and second stages as if their p-values will be combined according to the rule

$$p_{Combine} = \Phi\left(\frac{\Phi^{-1}(p_2) \cdot \sqrt{f_N} + \Phi^{-1}(p_3) \cdot \sqrt{f_{N_{Adapt}}}}{\sqrt{f_N + f_{N_{Adapt}}}}\right) \quad (15.2)$$

and the study will be considered positive if $p_{Combine} < 0.025$ or if

$$p_3 \leq \Phi\left(\frac{\Phi^{-1}(.025) \cdot \sqrt{f_N + f_{N\,Adapt}} - \Phi^{-1}(\alpha_2) \cdot \sqrt{f_N}}{\sqrt{f_{N\,Adapt}}}\right) \tag{15.3}$$

So, if both stages are passed successfully, then the significance of the result will be at least 0.025.

Let's consider what happens to the efficiency as $f_{N\,Adapt}$ decreases to f_N and z_{α_3} declines as a result from $z_{\alpha_3} = \Phi^{-1}(0.025)$ to $z_{\alpha_3} = \Phi^{-1}(.025) \cdot \sqrt{2} - \Phi^{-1}(\alpha_2)$. That is, we want to examine what happens when the Phase 2/3 program changes incrementally from a traditional two-study design toward an adaptive Phase 2/3 design where the size of the Phase 2 and Phase 3 components are the same. To do so, first we need to determine what happens to the optimal proportion of drugs that may provide clinical benefit, p, as $f_{N\,Adapt}$ changes. If p is such that the efficiency is optimized, then from the first derivative, $\partial \eta / \partial p$, we can deduce that

$$C + N\left[f_N + f_{N\,Adapt} \cdot \left(p \cdot \Phi\left(z_{\alpha_2} - [z_{\alpha_3} - z_\beta] \cdot f_\delta \cdot \sqrt{f_N}\right) + (1-p)\alpha_2\right)\right]$$
$$- p\left[f_{N\,Adapt} \cdot N\left(\Phi\left(z_{\alpha_2} - [z_{\alpha_3} - z_\beta] \cdot f_\delta \cdot \sqrt{f_N}\right) - \alpha_2\right) + \frac{\partial C}{\partial p}\right] = 0 \tag{15.4}$$

which is equivalent to

$$C(p) + N \cdot \left(f_N + f_{N\,Adapt}\alpha_2\right) - p \cdot \frac{\partial C}{\partial p} = 0 \tag{15.5}$$

and also

$$\frac{C(p) + N \cdot \left(f_N + f_{N\,Adapt}\alpha_2\right)}{p} = \frac{\partial C}{\partial p} \tag{15.6}$$

This equation can be interpreted as stating that the expected cost of failing per truly effective drug entering clinical development equals the marginal research cost of increasing the probability of a truly effective drug entering development.

This equation must be satisfied if the probability that a drug is truly effective at the start of clinical development, p, maximizes the efficiency. That is, if the amount of money spent to develop new molecules prior to entering clinical development is optimal. Now let's see what happens to this value of p when $f_{N\,Adapt}$ changes. Implicitly, differentiating Equation (15.5) with respect to $f_{N\,Adapt}$ leads to

$$\frac{\partial C(p)}{\partial p} \cdot \frac{\partial p}{\partial f_{N_{Adapt}}} + N \cdot \alpha_2 - \left[p \cdot \frac{\partial^2 C}{\partial p^2} \frac{\partial p}{\partial f_{N_{Adapt}}} + \frac{\partial p}{\partial f_{N_{Adapt}}} \frac{\partial C}{\partial p} \right] = 0 \qquad (15.7)$$

or

$$N \cdot \alpha_2 - p \cdot \frac{\partial^2 C}{\partial p^2} \frac{\partial p}{\partial f_{N_{Adapt}}} = 0 \qquad (15.8)$$

which further reduces to

$$\frac{\partial p}{\partial f_{N_{Adapt}}} = \frac{N \cdot \alpha_2}{p \cdot \dfrac{\partial^2 C}{\partial p^2}} \qquad (15.9)$$

Now since $\frac{\partial^2 C}{\partial p^2} > 0$, that is, to increase the probability of a successful molecule coming out of research takes ever increasing costs, $\frac{\partial p}{\partial f_{N_{Adapt}}} > 0$. Thus, reducing $f_{N_{Adapt}}$ and letting more Phase 2 data be used as part of the evidence accumulated in Phase 3 provides an incentive to drug and biotech companies to put more drugs into clinical development, drugs that on the margin have a lower probability of success. Alternatively, drug companies could spend less money on research for molecules that are going into clinical development and thereby reduce p.

15.2 Net Effect of Adaptive Phase 2/3 Designs on the Ratio of True to False Positives

Now we can ask how will this behavior induced by adaptive designs along with the direct effect on the critical value in Phase 3 change the ratio of true positives to false positives.

The ratio of true positives to false positives is

$$\frac{P(T,+)}{P(F,+)} = \frac{p \cdot \Phi\left(z_{\alpha_2} - \left[z_{\alpha_3} - z_\beta\right] \cdot f_\delta \cdot \sqrt{f_N}\right) \cdot \Phi\left(z_{\alpha_3} - \left[z_{\alpha_3} - z_\beta\right] \cdot f_\delta \cdot \sqrt{f_{N_{Adapt}}}\right)}{(1-p) \cdot \alpha_2 \cdot \alpha_3} \qquad (15.10)$$

Now when $f_{N_{adapt}}$ decreases, p must decrease to maximize efficiency, and we would expect α_3 to increase when α_2 is small and decrease when α_2 is large. Now let's formally evaluate the impact on the ratio of true to false positives. The derivative of the ratio of true to false positives with respect to $f_{N_{Adapt}}$ is

$$\frac{\partial}{\partial f_{N Adapt}} \frac{P(T,+)}{P(F,+)}$$

$$= \frac{\left[\begin{array}{l} \left[(1-p) \cdot \alpha_2 \cdot \alpha_3 \cdot \left(p \cdot \Phi(z_{\alpha_2}-\ldots) \cdot \dfrac{\partial \Phi(z_{\alpha_3*}-\ldots)}{\partial f_{N Adapt}} + \dfrac{\partial p}{\partial f_{N Adapt}} \Phi(z_{\alpha_2}-\ldots) \cdot \Phi(z_{\alpha_3*}-\ldots)\right)\right] \\ -p \cdot \Phi(z_{\alpha_2}-\ldots) \cdot \Phi(z_{\alpha_3*}-\ldots) \cdot \left((-1)\dfrac{\partial p}{\partial f_{N Adapt}} \cdot \alpha_2 \cdot \alpha_3 + (1-p) \cdot \alpha_2 \dfrac{\partial \alpha_3}{\partial f_{N Adapt}}\right) \end{array}\right]}{\left((1-p) \cdot \alpha_2 \cdot \alpha_3^*\right)^2}$$

(15.11)

$$= (1-p) \cdot \alpha_2 \cdot \alpha_3 \cdot p \cdot \Phi(z_{\alpha_2}-\ldots) \cdot \frac{\partial \Phi(z_{\alpha_3*}-\ldots)}{\partial f_{N Adapt}} \qquad (15.12)$$

$$+ \alpha_2 \cdot \alpha_3 \cdot \Phi(z_{\alpha_2}-\ldots) \cdot \Phi(z_{\alpha_3*}-\ldots) \cdot \frac{\partial p}{\partial f_{N Adapt}}$$

$$- p \cdot \Phi(z_{\alpha_2}-\ldots) \cdot \Phi(z_{\alpha_3*}-\ldots) \cdot (1-p) \cdot \alpha_2 \frac{\partial \alpha_3}{\partial f_{N Adapt}}$$

Now the coefficient of $\dfrac{\partial p}{\partial f_{N Adapt}}$ is greater than zero so the impact on the ratio of true to false positives of reducing $f_{N Adapt}$ mediated through p will be to reduce the ratio of true to false positives. To determine the net effect on the ratio of true to false positives, we also have to account for the other terms in the derivative, those involving $\dfrac{\partial \Phi\left(z_{\alpha_3*} - [z_{\alpha_3} - z_\beta] \cdot f_\delta \cdot \sqrt{f_{N Adapt}}\right)}{\partial f_{N Adapt}}$ and $\dfrac{\partial \alpha_3}{\partial f_{N Adapt}}$. The signs of the coefficients for these terms are positive and negative, respectively. Figures 15.1, 15.2, and 15.3 describe how these two terms on net change as $f_{N Adapt}$ changes with $f_\delta = 1$, 1.5, and 3.0. As noted earlier, $z_{\alpha_3^*}$ is a function of $f_{N Adapt}$.

If f_δ equals one then the net change in these two components of the derivative is positive for α_2 ranging from 0.05 to 0.50 one sided, values of α_2 that are commonly used in Phase 2 trials. So, in these circumstances the ratio of true to false positives will decrease when $f_{N Adapt}$ decreases. Thus, permitting adaptive designs to be used that reduce the total number of patients studied in a clinical program will reduce the ratio of true to false positives. On the other hand, if the treatment effect is larger than what is planned for in the Phase 3 trial (e.g., $f_\delta = 1.5$ or 3.0), then reducing $f_{N Adapt}$ may lead to an improved ratio of true to false positives if α_2 is in the range of 0.20 to 0.50 and if it is very difficult to increase the proportion of molecules entering clinical development that can ultimately help patients, that is, if $\dfrac{\partial p}{\partial f_{N Adapt}}$ is

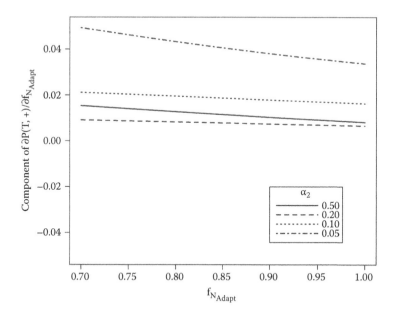

FIGURE 15.1

Component of the derivative of true positives/false positives with respect to $f_{N_{Adapt}}$, $f_\delta = 1$.

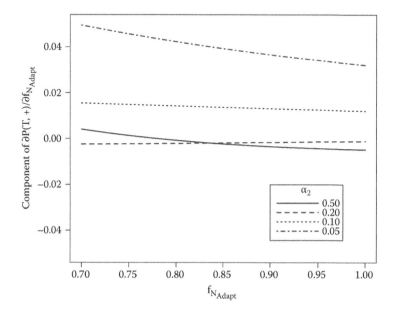

FIGURE 15.2

Component of the derivative of true positives/false positives with respect to $f_{N_{Adapt}}$, $f_\delta = 1.5$.

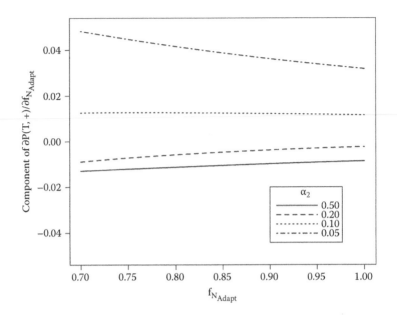

FIGURE 15.3
Component of the derivative of true positives/false positives with respect to $f_{N_{Adapt}}$, $f_8 = 3.0$.

close to zero. Thus, in most circumstances allowing companies to use more data from Phase 2 as part of the information that is required for an 80 to 90 percent powered Phase 3 trial will decrease the ratio of true to false positives. At the same time, the efficiency of drug development will increase.

Reference

Bauer, P. (1989). Multistage testing with adaptive designs: With discussion. *Biometrie und Informatik in Medizin und Biologie* 20:130–148.

16

Size of the Phase 3 Trial

Phase 3 trials are typically sized to have 80 to 90 percent power at a treatment effect size that represents the minimum clinically meaningful difference. Until this point, we have taken the Phase 3 sample size to be such a fixed known quantity at the beginning of a clinical trial program. In this section we assess whether increasing the Phase 3 sample size beyond these levels will improve the efficiency of drug development. We will also look at whether sizing the Phase 3 trial based on the results of Phase 2 can improve efficiency.

16.1 Sizing a Phase 3 Trial Based on the Minimum Clinically Meaningful Difference

Let's express the efficiency of a Phase 2/Phase 3 program as follows:

$$E = \frac{p \cdot \Phi\left(z_{\alpha_2} - \delta\sqrt{n_2}\right) \cdot \Phi\left(z_{\alpha_3} - \delta\sqrt{n_3}\right)}{C + n_2 + n_3 \cdot \left[p \cdot \Phi\left(z_{\alpha_2} - \delta\sqrt{n_2}\right) + (1-p) \cdot \alpha_2\right]} \tag{16.1}$$

We choose this representation for efficiency since the Phase 3 sample size is explicitly represented as n_3 instead of indirectly as f_{N3}.

With this representation for efficiency, $\partial E/\partial n_3$ will be greater than zero if

$$\left(C + n_2 + n_3 \cdot \left[p \cdot \Phi\left(z_{\alpha_2} - \delta\sqrt{n_2}\right) + (1-p) \cdot \alpha_2\right]\right) \times \phi\left(z_{\alpha_3} - \delta\sqrt{n_3}\right) \cdot \left(\frac{-\delta}{2}\right) \cdot n_3^{-1/2}$$

$$- \Phi\left(z_{\alpha_3} - \delta\sqrt{n_3}\right) \cdot \left[p \cdot \Phi\left(z_{\alpha_2} - \delta\sqrt{n_2}\right) + (1-p) \cdot \alpha_2\right] > 0 \tag{16.2}$$

or

$$\frac{C+n_2}{n_3} \cdot \phi\left(z_{\alpha_3} - \delta\sqrt{n_3}\right) \cdot \left(\frac{-\delta}{2}\right) \cdot \sqrt{n_3}$$

$$+ \left[p \cdot \Phi\left(z_{\alpha_2} - \delta\sqrt{n_2}\right) + (1-p) \cdot \alpha_2\right] \cdot \begin{bmatrix} \phi\left(z_{\alpha_3} - \delta\sqrt{n_3}\right) \cdot \left(\frac{-\delta}{2}\right)\sqrt{n_3} \\ -\Phi\left(z_{\alpha_3} - \delta\sqrt{n_3}\right) \end{bmatrix} > 0 \tag{16.3}$$

or finally

$$p \cdot \Phi\left(z_{\alpha_2} - \delta\sqrt{n_2}\right) + (1-p) \cdot \alpha_2 < \frac{(C+n_2)/n_3 \cdot \phi\left(z_{\alpha_3} - \delta\sqrt{n_3}\right) \cdot (\delta/2)\sqrt{n_3}}{\phi\left(z_{\alpha_3} - \delta\sqrt{n_3}\right) \cdot (-\delta/2)\sqrt{n_3} - \Phi\left(z_{\alpha_3} - \delta\sqrt{n_3}\right)}$$

(16.4)

since

$$\phi\left(z_{\alpha_3} - \delta\sqrt{n_3}\right) \cdot \left(\frac{-\delta}{2}\right)\sqrt{n_3} - \Phi\left(z_{\alpha_3} - \delta\sqrt{n_3}\right) < 0$$

(16.5)

for $\delta < 0$, which can be seen by graphing $\Phi\left(z_{\alpha_3} - x\right) \cdot \left(\frac{-x}{2}\right) - \Phi\left(z_{\alpha_3} - x\right)$ for $x < 0$.

If the trial is powered at 80 percent with a type 1 error of 0.025, then

$$\phi\left(z_{\alpha_3} - \delta\sqrt{n_3}\right) = 0.28$$

(16.6)

$$\Phi\left(z_{\alpha_3} - \delta\sqrt{n_3}\right) = 0.80$$

(16.7)

$$\left(-\frac{\delta}{2}\right)\sqrt{n_3} = 1.40$$

(16.8)

So, the Phase 3 sample size should be increased if

$$p \cdot \Phi\left(z_{\alpha_2} - \delta\sqrt{n_2}\right) + (1-p) \cdot \alpha_2 < \frac{(C+n_2)/n_3 \cdot 0.28 \cdot (-1.4)}{0.28 \cdot (1.4) - 0.80}$$

(16.9)

$$= (C + n_2)/n_3 \cdot 0.96$$

(16.10)

That is, if the Phase 2 trial is such that the chance of moving forward to Phase 3 is less than $(C + n_2)/n_3 \cdot 0.96$, then the change in efficiency with respect to n_3 is greater than zero, which means efficiency is improved by increasing the Phase 3 sample size. On the other hand, if the chance of moving forward to Phase 3 is greater than $(C + n_2)/n_3 \cdot 0.96$, then the change in efficiency with respect to n_3 is less than zero and one should conduct the 80 percent powered trial, which is the smallest trial one can conduct in Phase 3 and hope to gain regulatory approval. If we are developing a new molecule, we would expect

C to be about the same size as n_3 and so the size of the Phase 3 trial should be increased beyond what it would be for an 80 percent powered trial.

16.2 Using Phase 2 Results to Size the Phase 3 Trial

An alternative approach to sizing a trial based on the minimum clinically meaningful difference is to size it based on the treatment effect observed in Phase 2. Here, we will evaluate the efficiency of sizing the Phase 3 trial in this way.

The estimate of the treatment effect from a randomized Phase 2 can be described as

$$\frac{\bar{X}_T - \bar{X}_T}{\sqrt{2 \cdot s^2}} \approx N\left(\frac{\mu_T - \mu_T}{\sqrt{2 \cdot \sigma^2}}, 1/n_2\right) = N(\delta, 1/n_2) \tag{16.11}$$

The Phase 3 sample size based on this estimate of the treatment effect would be

$$n_3 = \frac{(z_{\alpha_3} + z_\beta)^2}{\delta^2} \tag{16.12}$$

The efficiency of a strategy that determines the Phase 3 sample size in this way can then be written as

$$\frac{p \cdot \Phi\left(z_{\alpha_2} - \delta\sqrt{n_2}\right) \cdot \dfrac{\displaystyle\int_{-\infty}^{\frac{z_{\alpha_2}}{\sqrt{n_2}}} \Phi\left(z_{\alpha_3} - \delta\sqrt{n_3(\Delta)}\right) \cdot \phi\left([\Delta - \delta] \cdot \sqrt{n_2}\right) \cdot \sqrt{n_2} \cdot d\Delta}{\displaystyle\int_{-\infty}^{\frac{z_{\alpha_2}}{\sqrt{n_2}}} \phi\left([\Delta - \delta] \cdot \sqrt{n_2}\right) \cdot \sqrt{n_2} \cdot d\Delta}}{C + n_2 + (z_{\alpha_3} + z_\beta)^2 \cdot \dfrac{\displaystyle\int_{-\infty}^{\frac{z_{\alpha_2}}{\sqrt{n_2}}} 1/\Delta^2 \cdot \phi\left([\Delta - \delta] \cdot \sqrt{n_2}\right) \cdot \sqrt{n_2} \cdot d\Delta}{\displaystyle\int_{-\infty}^{\frac{z_{\alpha_2}}{\sqrt{n_2}}} \phi\left([\Delta - \delta] \cdot \sqrt{n_2}\right) \cdot \sqrt{n_2} \cdot d\Delta} \cdot \left(p \cdot \Phi\left(z_{\alpha_2} - \delta\sqrt{n_2}\right) + (1 - p) \cdot \alpha_2\right)}$$

$$\tag{16.13}$$

Here, Δ represents the true value of the treatment effect. In the numerator we have replaced the power in Phase 3 with the expected power and in the denominator we replaced the Phase 3 sample size with the expected sample size, all accounting for the fact that Phase 3 is only undertaken if the Phase 2 Z-statistic is such that $Z < z_{\alpha_2}$.

Figure 16.1 presents the efficiency for five scenarios: one just for comparison purposes where the Phase 3 sample size provides 80 percent power at every δ; one where the Phase 3 sample yields 80 percent power at the treatment effect observed in Phase 2; and finally, three where the Phase 3 sample size is based on a treatment effect size of 0.10, 0.15, and 0.20. C, which represents pre-Phase 2 development costs, is taken to be zero. The Phase 2 sample size is 50 subjects per group. The solid line represents the efficiency when the Phase 3 trial is sized based on the treatment effect observed in Phase 2. This approach results in the greatest efficiency of all the approaches presented in Figure 16.1. This is not the case, however, when the pre-Phase 2 development costs, C, are greater than zero, as is illustrated in Figure 16.2. In Figure 16.2 we see that the approach of sizing the Phase 3 trial based on the Phase 2 results is not uniformly better than the other approaches presented in the figure. That is, when there are considerable pre-Phase 2 development costs to account for, sizing a Phase 3 trial based on the treatment effect size observed in Phase 2 can actually reduce the efficiency of drug development. An approach where the sample size is chosen so that the study is powered to detect a clinically meaningful treatment effect could yield greater efficiency, as in the case of δ = 0.15 and δ = 0.20 in Figure 16.2.

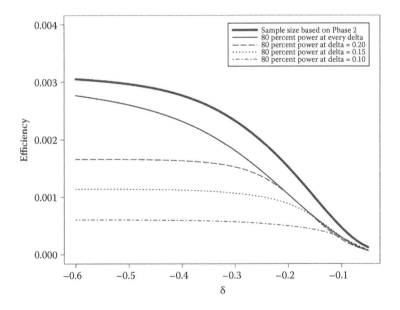

FIGURE 16.1
Efficiency of approaches to determining the Phase 3 sample size. C = 0.

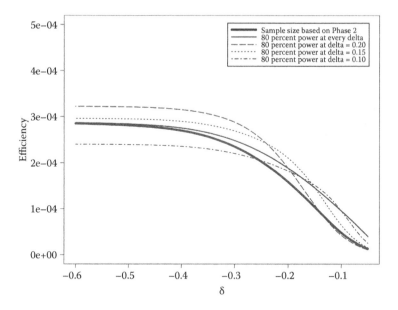

FIGURE 16.2
Efficiency of approaches to determining the Phase 3 sample size. $C = 500$.

17

Extending the Model of Clinical Drug Development

Until this point, we have focused primarily on maximizing the efficiency of a clinical development program that is comprised of a Phase 2 screening trial followed by an 80 percent powered Phase 3 trial with a single analysis at completion. In this chapter we extend the model of clinical development in three ways. First, we look at the model from the point of view of maximizing net present value (NPV) when the project is part of a portfolio of other projects. Second, we consider a model of clinical development where the Phase 2 trial is designed to pick the better of two doses to go forward to Phase 3 and the Phase 3 trial includes an interim analysis. And finally, we consider a model of drug development for studying new molecules that may have enhanced activity in a subpopulation with high expression of a specific marker.

17.1 Maximizing Net Present Value (NPV)

As we noted in Chapter 2, optimizing a clinical development program in a way that maximizes NPV when the drug under consideration is just one of many other drugs in a product portfolio involves selecting the parameters of the Phase 2 trial such that Equations (17.1) through (17.5) are satisfied.

$$PV_1 + \lambda \cdot \text{Cost}_1 = 0 \tag{17.1}$$

$$\frac{\partial PV_1}{\partial \alpha_{2,1}} + \lambda \cdot \frac{\partial \text{Cost}_1}{\partial \alpha_{2,1}} = 0 \tag{17.2}$$

$$\frac{\partial PV_1}{\partial fN_{2,1}} + \lambda \cdot \frac{\partial \text{Cost}_1}{\partial fN_{2,1}} = 0 \tag{17.3}$$

$$\frac{\partial PV_2}{\partial \alpha_{2,2}} + \lambda \cdot \frac{\partial \text{Cost}_2}{\partial \alpha_{2,2}} = 0 \tag{17.4}$$

$$\frac{\partial PV_2}{\partial fN_{2,2}} + \lambda \cdot \frac{\partial \text{Cost}_2}{\partial fN_{2,2}} = 0 \tag{17.5}$$

Here, PV_1 denotes the present value of the expected future cash flows from the project in the portfolio with the smallest present value and represents the increase in the present value of the company's future cash flows from adding another drug into clinical development. PV_2 represents the present value of the expected future cash flows from the project whose Phase 2 study design we wish to optimize so as to maximize NPV of the company. In terms of the model of drug development we have previously set forth, the optimal design of the Phase 2 trial for project 2 is determined by Equations (17.6) through (17.10):

$$\lambda = \frac{PV_1 \cdot p \cdot \Phi\left(z_{\alpha_{2,1}} - \left[z_{\alpha_3} - z_\beta\right] \cdot f_\delta \cdot \sqrt{f_{N_{2,1}}}\right) \cdot \Phi\left(z_{\alpha_3} - \left[z_{\alpha_3} - z_\beta\right] \cdot f_\delta\right)}{f_{N_{2,1}} + p \cdot \Phi\left(z_{\alpha_{2,1}} - \left[z_{\alpha_3} - z_\beta\right] \cdot f_\delta \cdot \sqrt{f_{N_{2,1}}}\right) + (1 - p) \cdot \alpha_{2,1}} \tag{17.6}$$

$$\lambda = \frac{PV_1 \cdot \partial\left[p \cdot \Phi\left(z_{\alpha_{2,1}} - \left[z_{\alpha_3} - z_\beta\right] \cdot f_\delta \cdot \sqrt{f_{N_{2,1}}}\right) \cdot \Phi\left(z_{\alpha_3} - \left[z_{\alpha_3} - z_\beta\right] \cdot f_\delta\right)\right] / \partial \alpha_{2,1}}{\partial\left[f_{N_{2,1}} + p \cdot \Phi\left(z_{\alpha_{2,1}} - \left[z_{\alpha_3} - z_\beta\right] \cdot f_\delta \cdot \sqrt{f_{N_{2,1}}}\right) + (1 - p) \cdot \alpha_{2,1}\right] / \partial \alpha_{2,1}}$$

$$\tag{17.7}$$

$$\lambda = \frac{PV_2 \cdot \partial\left[p \cdot \Phi\left(z_{\alpha_{2,2}} - \left[z_{\alpha_3} - z_\beta\right] \cdot f_\delta \cdot \sqrt{f_{N_{2,2}}}\right) \cdot \Phi\left(z_{\alpha_3} - \left[z_{\alpha_3} - z_\beta\right] \cdot f_\delta\right)\right] / \partial \alpha_{2,2}}{\partial\left[f_{N_{2,2}} + p \cdot \Phi\left(z_{\alpha_{2,2}} - \left[z_{\alpha_3} - z_\beta\right] \cdot f_\delta \cdot \sqrt{f_{N_{2,2}}}\right) + (1 - p) \cdot \alpha_{2,2}\right] / \partial \alpha_{2,2}}$$

$$\tag{17.8}$$

$$\lambda = \frac{PV_1 \cdot \partial\left[p \cdot \Phi\left(z_{\alpha_{2,1}} - \left[z_{\alpha_3} - z_\beta\right] \cdot f_\delta \cdot \sqrt{f_{N_{2,1}}}\right) \cdot \Phi\left(z_{\alpha_3} - \left[z_{\alpha_3} - z_\beta\right] \cdot f_\delta\right)\right] / \partial f_{N_{2,1}}}{\partial\left[f_{N_{2,1}} + p \cdot \Phi\left(z_{\alpha_{2,1}} - \left[z_{\alpha_3} - z_\beta\right] \cdot f_\delta \cdot \sqrt{f_{N_{2,1}}}\right) + (1 - p) \cdot \alpha_{2,1}\right] / \partial f_{N_{2,1}}}$$

$$\tag{17.9}$$

$$\lambda = \frac{PV_2 \cdot \partial\left[p \cdot \Phi\left(z_{\alpha_{2,2}} - \left[z_{\alpha_3} - z_\beta\right] \cdot f_\delta \cdot \sqrt{f_{N_{2,2}}}\right) \cdot \Phi\left(z_{\alpha_3} - \left[z_{\alpha_3} - z_\beta\right] \cdot f_\delta\right)\right] / \partial f_{N_{2,2}}}{\partial\left[f_{N_{2,2}} + p \cdot \Phi\left(z_{\alpha_{2,2}} - \left[z_{\alpha_3} - z_\beta\right] \cdot f_\delta \cdot \sqrt{f_{N_{2,2}}}\right) + (1 - p) \cdot \alpha_{2,2}\right] / \partial f_{N_{2,2}}}$$

$$\tag{17.10}$$

Here, in Equations (17.6) through (17.10), PV_1 and PV_2 simply represent the present value of expected future cash flows assuming the project was successful. In Equations (17.1) through (17.5) they also accounted for the probability of technical success, that is, the probability of a successful development all the way through to a positive Phase 3 trial. In addition, $z_{\alpha_2,i}$ represents the critical value in Phase 2 for project i and $f_{N2,i}$ represents the sample size of the Phase 2 trial for project i as a fraction of the sample size in Phase 3 that would provide 80 percent power. Note that we are assuming the costs are the same for Project 1 and Project 2. However, without loss of generality we could incorporate costs into PV_1 and PV_2 by letting them instead represent $PV/Cost$. Equations (17.6) through (17.10) imply that

$$\frac{\partial\Big[\, p\cdot\Phi\big(z_{\alpha_{2,2}}-[z_{\alpha_3}-z_\beta]\cdot f_\delta\cdot\sqrt{f_{N_2}}\big)\cdot\Phi\big(z_{\alpha_3}-[z_{\alpha_3}-z_\beta]\cdot f_\delta\big)\Big]/\partial\alpha_{2,2}}{\partial\Big[\,f_{N_2}+p\cdot\Phi\big(z_{\alpha_{2,2}}-[z_{\alpha_3}-z_\beta]\cdot f_\delta\cdot\sqrt{f_{N_2}}\big)+(1-p)\cdot\alpha_{2,2}\,\Big]/\partial\alpha_{2,2}}\cdot\frac{PV2}{PV1}$$

$$(17.11)$$

$$=\frac{\partial\Big[\, p\cdot\Phi\big(z_{\alpha_{2,1}}-[z_{\alpha_3}-z_\beta]\cdot f_\delta\cdot\sqrt{f_{N_1}}\big)\cdot\Phi\big(z_{\alpha_3}-[z_{\alpha_3}-z_\beta]\cdot f_\delta\big)\Big]/\partial\alpha_{2,1}}{\partial\Big[\,f_{N_1}+p\cdot\Phi\big(z_{\alpha_{2,1}}-[z_{\alpha_3}-z_\beta]\cdot f_\delta\cdot\sqrt{f_{N_1}}\big)+(1-p)\cdot\alpha_{2,1}\,\Big]/\partial\alpha_{2,1}}$$

$$(17.12)$$

$$=\frac{p\cdot\Phi\big(z_{\alpha_{2,1}}-[z_{\alpha_3}-z_\beta]\cdot f_\delta\cdot\sqrt{f_{N_1}}\big)\cdot\Phi\big(z_{\alpha_3}-[z_{\alpha_3}-z_\beta]\cdot f_\delta\big)}{f_{N_1}+p\cdot\Phi\big(z_{\alpha_{21}}-[z_{\alpha_3}-z_\beta]\cdot f_\delta\cdot\sqrt{f_{N_1}}\big)+(1-p)\cdot\alpha_{2,1}}$$

$$(17.13)$$

and similarly

$$\frac{\partial\Big[\, p\cdot\Phi\big(z_{\alpha_{2,2}}-[z_{\alpha_3}-z_\beta]\cdot f_\delta\cdot\sqrt{f_{N_2}}\big)\cdot\Phi\big(z_{\alpha_3}-[z_{\alpha_3}-z_\beta]\cdot f_\delta\big)\Big]/\partial f_{N_2}}{\partial\Big[\,f_{N_2}+p\cdot\Phi\big(z_{\alpha_{2,2}}-[z_{\alpha_3}-z_\beta]\cdot f_\delta\cdot\sqrt{f_{N_2}}\big)+(1-p)\cdot\alpha_{2,2}\,\Big]/\partial f_{N_2}}\cdot\frac{PV_2}{PV_1}$$

$$(17.14)$$

$$=\frac{p\cdot\Phi\big(z_{\alpha_{2,1}}-[z_{\alpha_3}-z_\beta]\cdot f_\delta\cdot\sqrt{f_{N_1}}\big)\cdot\Phi\big(z_{\alpha_3}-[z_{\alpha_3}-z_\beta]\cdot f_\delta\big)}{f_{N_1}+p\cdot\Phi\big(z_{\alpha_{2,1}}-[z_{\alpha_3}-z_\beta]\cdot f_\delta\cdot\sqrt{f_{N_1}}\big)+(1-p)\cdot\alpha_{2,1}}$$

$$(17.15)$$

Equations (17.11) through (17.15) provide a way to determine the design of a Phase 2 trial that will maximize the present value of expected future cash flows per investment and *a fortiori* NPV. First, the Phase 2 study design that maximizes efficiency has to be determined along with the associated level of efficiency. Then the design that maximizes NPV will be the design where the change in the expected number of successful Phase 3 trials divided by the change in the cost when changing either α_2 or f_{N2} times the ratio of the present value of expected cash flows for project 2 to project 1 equals the maximum efficiency. Alternatively, one could say that the changes in the present value of expected future cash flows due to changes in α_2 and f_{N2} must be the same as the change in present value from adding a new study to clinical development. These changes in present value are relative to the changes in cost incurred as represented by the change in expected sample size of clinical development for changes in α_2 and f_{N2}, and the expected sample size of a clinical development program for adding a new study.

Figure 17.1 and Figure 17.2 present the optimum program as a function of f_δ for a range of values for PV_2/PV_1. Figure 17.1 assumes that there are no

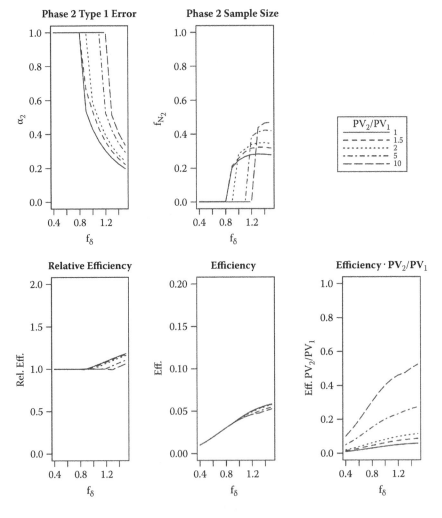

FIGURE 17.1
Phase 2 design that maximizes present value, pre-Phase 2 costs equal Phase 3 costs.

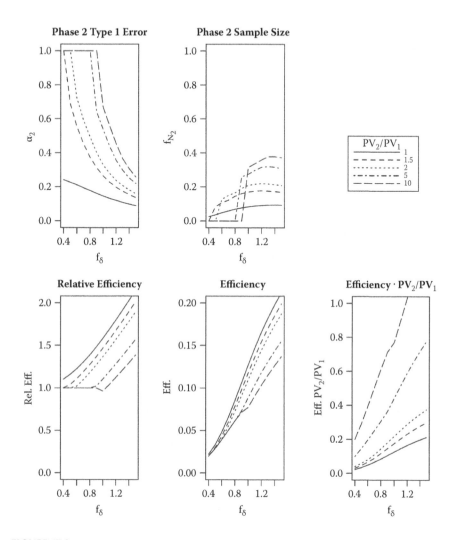

FIGURE 17.2
Phase 2 design that maximizes present value, pre-Phase 2 costs equal zero.

pre-Phase 2 costs, whereas Figure 17.2 assumes that there are pre-Phase 2 costs and that they are approximately equal to the Phase 3 costs.

As the ratio PV_2/PV_1 increases, the range of f_δ where $\alpha_2 = 1$ and $f_{N_2} = 0$, that is, where the optimal program does not include a Phase 2 trial, increases. Further, if a Phase 2 trial is warranted, as PV_2/PV_1 increases α_2 increases as well, making it more likely development will proceed from Phase 2 to Phase 3 to take advantage of the greater payoff if the drug is indeed effective. It is interesting to note that the efficiency does not change much unless PV_2/PV_1 is quite large.

If project 2 with the higher PV were designed instead so that it maximized efficiency, then the present value of the company could be increased by increasing α_2 and increasing f_{N_2} and reducing the number of molecules in development since these two actions increase the present value due to the studies underway more than the present value would be reduced by taking away studies from development.

Finally, note that in Figure 17.2, where it is assumed that there are no pre-Phase 2 costs, there is a big decrease in the efficiency as the ratio PV_2/PV_1 increases. So in these circumstances there is a cost to maximizing NPV based on uncertain information related to the cash flows generated by a successful drug project.

17.2 Picking the Best Dose in Phase 2

A common drug development strategy is to use the Phase 2 study to pick the best dose to evaluate in Phase 3, and then design the Phase 3 trial with a rejection and futility boundary to permit the study to stop early if the drug is more or less effective than anticipated. Here, we evaluate this sort of strategy to determine what the optimal designs are for the Phase 2 and Phase 3 trials. For the Phase 2 trial we assume two comparisons are made. The first is between the two active doses to see which dose has the best outcome. And the second is between the best dose and control. For the Phase 3 trial we assume that there is one interim analysis where the trial can be stopped for efficacy or for futility.

If we let $\bar{X}_0$, $\bar{X}_1$, and $\bar{X}_2$ represent the mean outcome for control and dose 1 and 2, respectively, with means θ_i and variances σ_i^2 then we can write the probability that dose 1 is greater than dose 2 as well as greater than the placebo as follows. First, note that the power of a Z-test for the difference in means between dose 1 and control given the mean for dose 1 can be written as

$$P\left(\frac{\bar{X}_1 - \bar{X}_0}{\sqrt{\sigma_1^2 + \sigma_0^2}} < z_{\alpha_2} \mid \bar{X}_1\right) = P\left(\frac{\bar{X}_0 - \theta_0}{\sigma_0} > \frac{\bar{X}_1 - z_{\alpha_2}\sqrt{\sigma_1^2 + \sigma_0^2} - \theta_0}{\sigma_0} \mid \bar{X}_1\right) \quad (17.16)$$

$$= 1 - \Phi\left(\frac{\bar{X}_1 - \theta_1}{\sigma_1} \cdot \sqrt{\frac{\sigma_1^2}{\sigma_0^2}} - z_{\alpha_2} \cdot \sqrt{\frac{\sigma_1^2 + \sigma_0^2}{\sigma_0^2}} + \frac{\theta_1 - \theta_0}{\sqrt{\sigma_1^2 + \sigma_0^2}} \cdot \sqrt{\frac{\sigma_1^2 + \sigma_0^2}{\sigma_0^2}}\right) \quad (17.17)$$

We will assume that $\sigma_0^2 = \sigma_1^2$, so the preceding equation simplifies to

$$1 - \Phi\left(z - \sqrt{2} \cdot z_{\alpha_2} + \sqrt{2} \cdot \frac{\theta_1 - \theta_0}{\sqrt{2 \cdot \sigma^2}}\right) \quad (17.18)$$

Here, z is an observation from a standard normal distribution. Since the event $\bar{X}_1$ is less than $\bar{X}_2$ and the event $\bar{X}_1$ is less than $\bar{X}_0$ are independent given the value of $\bar{X}_1$, we can write the probability of the intersection of these two events as

$$\int_{-\infty}^{\infty} \left\{ \begin{array}{l} \left[1 - \Phi\left(z - \sqrt{2} \cdot z_{\alpha_2} + \sqrt{2} \cdot \left(z_{\alpha_3} - z_\beta \right) \cdot \sqrt{f_N} \cdot f_{\delta_1} \right) \right] \\ \times \left[1 - \Phi\left(z + \sqrt{2} \cdot \left(z_{\alpha_3} - z_\beta \right) \cdot \sqrt{f_N} \cdot \left(f_{\delta_1} - f_{\delta_2} \right) \right) \right] \end{array} \right\} \cdot \phi(z) \cdot dz \quad (17.19)$$

We dropped the term $\sqrt{2} \cdot z_{\alpha_2}$ in the second term of the product in Equation (17.19) since we are just looking to see if dose 1 has a greater mean than dose 2, that is, $\alpha_2 = 0.50$ and $z_{\alpha_2} = 0$.

If we denote this probability by $wt(\alpha_2, \alpha_3, \beta, f_{\delta_1}, f_{\delta_2}, f_n)$, then we can write the efficiency of drug development as

$$\frac{p \cdot \left[\begin{array}{l} wt(\alpha_2, \alpha_3, \beta, f_{\delta_1}, f_{\delta_2}, 2/3 \cdot f_N) \cdot P(+\text{Ph3, Dose 1}) \\ \\ + wt(\alpha_2, \alpha_3, \beta, f_{\delta_2}, f_{\delta_1}, 2/3 \cdot f_N) \cdot P(+\text{Ph3, Dose 2}) \end{array} \right]}{\left\{ \begin{array}{l} \left[1 + f_n + p \cdot \left[wt(\alpha_2, \alpha_3, \beta, f_{\delta_1}, f_{\delta_2}, 2/3 \cdot f_N) \cdot E(f_{N_1}) \right. \right. \\ \\ \left. \left. + wt(\alpha_2, \alpha_3, \beta, f_{\delta_2}, f_{\delta_1}, 2/3 \cdot f_N) \cdot E(f_{N_2}) \right] \right] \\ \\ + (1-p) \cdot wt(\alpha_2, \alpha_3, \beta, 0, 0, 2/3 \cdot f_N) \cdot E(f_{N_0}) \end{array} \right\}} \quad (17.20)$$

Here, $P(+\text{Ph3, Dose 1})$ is the probability of a successful Phase 3 when dose 1 is used and $P(+\text{Ph3, Dose 2})$ is the probability of a successful Phase 3 trial when dose 2 is used. $2/3 \cdot f_N$ represents the fraction of N used in the two-group comparison.

As noted earlier, we introduced an interim analysis into the Phase 3 trial for this development strategy. Here, $E(f_{N_1})$ and $E(f_{N_2})$ are the expected sample sizes for the Phase 3 trial when the treatment effect sizes are δ_1 and δ_2, respectively. $E(f_{N_0})$ is the expected sample size under the null hypothesis of no treatment effect. $E(f_{N_i})$ can be thought of as dependent on the following parameters. The size of the study at the first interim analysis expressed as a fraction of the nominal Phase 3 sample size, f_{n_1}, the size of the study following the first interim analysis as a fraction of the nominal Phase 3 sample size, f_{n_2}, the futility boundary at the interim analysis, $ftbd$; the rejection boundary at the interim, $rjbd$; and the power of the trial, β. We are assuming that the rejection boundary at the final analysis is chosen so that the type 1 error for the study as a whole is 0.025 and that the power for the trial is β percent when the treatment effect is represented by $f_\delta = 1$. We can write $E(f_{N_i})$ to show these dependencies as

$$E(f_{N_i})_{[f_{n_1}, f_{n_2}, ftbd, rjbd, \alpha_3, \beta]} \quad (17.21)$$

The problem of optimizing the efficiency is thus one of maximizing Equation (17.20) over the parameters $f_N, \alpha_2, f_{n_1}, f_{n_2}, ftbd$, and $rjbd$ subject to the constraint that the Phase 3 trial has type 1 error of α_3 and power equal to β. Figure 17.3 shows the results of a numerical maximization of efficiency with regard to these parameters. Here, f_{δ_1} is assumed to equal one and f_{δ_0} is allowed to vary between zero and one. In addition, the pre-Phase 2 development costs are assumed to equal the Phase 3 costs.

It is interesting to note how the optimal Phase 2 design changes as the magnitude of f_{δ_0}, the treatment effect of the inferior dose, changes. If f_{δ_0} is zero meaning that the dose finding is comparing a no effect dose with a fully active dose, then the optimal Phase 2 sample size is 20 to 30 percent of the nominal Phase 3 sample size and the optimal Phase 2 critical value for comparing the best dose with control ranges from 0 to 0.75. As the magnitude of the treatment effect of the suboptimal dose increases to the magnitude of the full effect dose, then the optimal Phase 2 sample size approaches zero and the optimal critical value increases beyond 3. That is, it is not worthwhile to conduct a Phase 2 trial if one is confident that the dose chosen is nearly optimal. This may be the case with the development of antibodies in oncology where the targets are in similar tissues and the type of molecule has similar pharmacokinetics across a variety of different biologic targets. If there is not a lot of confidence in what the correct dose is, then one should use a considerable number of subjects studying dose in Phase 2. For example, if the Phase 3 trial is anticipated to enroll 400 subjects per group, then the Phase 2 trial may enroll up to 120 patients per group, which represents a value for f_{N_2} of 0.30.

It is also interesting to note in Figure 17.3 that the design of the Phase 3 study does not change much at all with the size of the treatment effect in the suboptimal dose. And further, that the properties of the Phase 3 trial are good for establishing the drug is effective, with a ratio of power to type 1 error at the final and interim analyses greater than 32. There is some inflation of type 1 error given full enrollment with a value of 0.06 one sided.

Figure 17.3 was constructed by calculating efficiency under the assumption that pre-Phase 2 development costs equal Phase 3 costs. Figure 17.4 illustrates the results from optimizing efficiency when these costs are taken to be zero, as in the case where a drug has already received its initial approval and the objective is to investigate new indications for the drug. That is, the pre-Phase 2 development costs have already been covered by its successful development in its initial indication.

The Phase 2 trial design in this case is much different than the Phase 2 trial design when pre-Phase 2 costs are incorporated into the calculation of efficiency. The sample size for the Phase 2 trial is not more than 20 percent of the Phase 3 trial size, and the critical value for the Z-test is approximately –1. In this case, the Phase 2 trial is being used to determine whether to go forward to do a Phase 3 trial, whereas in the previous case the Phase 2 trial was being used primarily to select the best dose to take

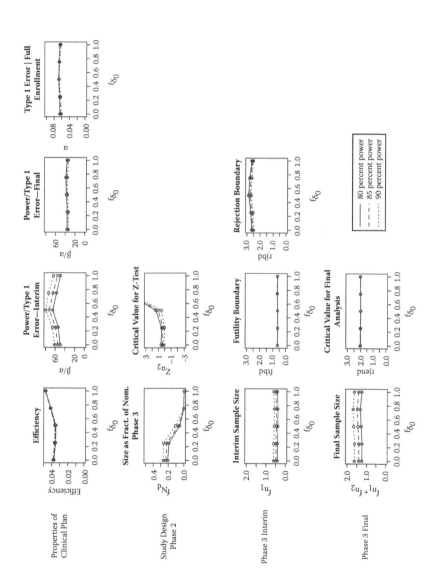

FIGURE 17.3
Properties of dose finding clinical plan, pre-Phase 2 development costs equal Phase 3 costs.

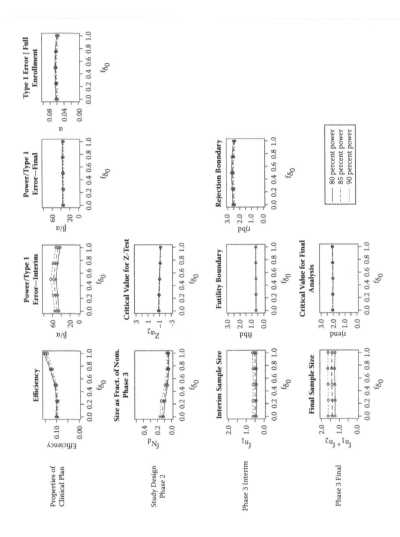

FIGURE 17.4

Properties of dose finding clinical plan, pre-Phase 2 development costs equal zero.

forward to Phase 3. Once again, the design of the Phase 3 trial does not change much as the magnitude of f_{δ_0}, the treatment effect of the inferior dose, changes.

Next we incorporate a second criteria in the Phase 2 decision for whether to go forward to Phase 3. That is, using oncology as an example, we incorporate rules related to progression-free survival (PFS) as well as to survival for judging which dose is the best, and then whether the best dose is better than the plaebo. To incorporate PFS, we just need to modify the expression for the probability of starting a Phase 3 trial and add an assumption about the probability that the drug has an effect on PFS when there is no effect on survival. The probability that the Phase 2 trial will support starting a Phase 3 trial based on PFS is

$$
\int_{-\infty}^{\infty}
\left[
\begin{array}{l}
\left[1 - \Phi\left(z - \sqrt{2} \cdot z_{\alpha_2} + \sqrt{2} \cdot \left(z_{\alpha_3} - z_\beta\right) \cdot \sqrt{f_N \cdot f_{n,pfs}} \cdot f_{\delta_1} \cdot f_{\delta,pfs}\right)\right] \\
\times \left[1 - \Phi\left(z + \sqrt{2} \cdot \left(z_{\alpha_3} - z_\beta\right) \cdot \sqrt{f_N \cdot f_{n,pfs}} \cdot \left(f_{\delta_1} - f_{\delta_2}\right) \cdot f_{\delta,pfs}\right)\right] \cdot \phi(z)
\end{array}
\right] \cdot dz
$$

$$(17.22)$$

Here, $f_{n,pfs}$ represents the percent increase in PFS events that are observed compared with deaths and $f_{\delta,pfs}$ represents the percent increase in the treatment effect in going from survival to PFS.

The probability that dose 1 passes the criteria based on PFS described in Equation (17.22) and meets the criteria based on survival is modeled as

$$
\int_{-\infty}^{\infty}
\left[
\begin{array}{l}
\left[1 - \Phi\left(z - \sqrt{2} \cdot z_{\alpha_{2PFS}} + \sqrt{2} \cdot \left(z_{\alpha_3} - z_\beta\right) \cdot \sqrt{f_N \cdot f_{n,pfs}} \cdot f_{\delta_1} \cdot f_{\delta,pfs}\right)\right] \\
\times \left[1 - \Phi\left(z + \sqrt{2} \cdot \left(z_{\alpha_3} - z_\beta\right) \cdot \sqrt{f_N \cdot f_{n,pfs}} \cdot \left(f_{\delta_1} - f_{\delta_2}\right) \cdot f_{\delta,pfs}\right)\right] \\
\times \Phi\left(z_{\alpha_{2Surv}} - \left(z_{\alpha_3} - z_\beta\right) \cdot f_{\delta_1} \cdot \sqrt{f_N}\right) \cdot \phi(z)
\end{array}
\right] \cdot dz
$$

$$(17.23)$$

Here, the first two terms are as in Equation (17.22). It is assumed that conditional on the null or the alternative, the probabilities associated with survival and progression are independent. We make a similar substitution in the expression for the probability that dose 2 passes the criteria to be studied in Phase 3.

The probability that the drug has an effect on PFS and not on survival is incorporated in the weight associated with the expected sample size for the

Phase 3 study under the null. Specifically, the weight associated with the expected sample size $E(f_{N_0})$ is now

$$(1 - p_{PFS}) \cdot wt(\alpha_2, \alpha_3, \beta, 0, 0, f_n) + p_{PFS} \cdot wt(\alpha_2, \alpha_3, \beta, f_{\delta_1} \cdot f_{\delta, pfs}, f_{\delta_2} \cdot f_{\delta, pfs}, f_n \cdot f_{n, pfs})$$

$$(17.24)$$

where p_{PFS} is the probability of a treatment effect on PFS under the null hypothesis.

Figures 17.5, 17.6, and 17.7 evaluate the clinical strategy when the probability of no effect on PFS under the null is 0.5, 0.7, and 0.9, respectively. We can see from the figures that as the probability of no effect on PFS under the null of no survival benefit increases, the critical value for the Z-test on PFS becomes stricter (more negative). Although the critical value for the Z-test in Phase 2 based on survival was negative when we did not consider PFS, the critical value when we do consider PFS in the Phase 2 go/no-go decision is positive. So, Phase 3 is undertaken if the active arm shows an improvement in PFS with no substantial worsening in survival compared to control.

17.3 Targeted Therapies

Herceptin was the first biologic that was successfully developed as a targeted therapy. When one reviews the development of Herceptin one sees that there was a great deal of science backing the idea that breast cancers that are HER2 positive are much more aggressive than those that are HER2 negative. There was even good scientific rationale for the idea that HER2 receptor activation is a direct growth stimulant for the disease and hence a good target for biologic therapies. Targeted therapies developed today typically do not have such a strong scientific basis as Herceptin did for working only in a population that expresses a particular marker. Indeed, at the start of clinical drug development it is usually an open question whether the drug will be effective in all subjects or only in those expressing a particular marker. Here, we will consider a three-stage strategy for the clinical evaluation of a drug and its potential marker. In the first stage, the drug is evaluated for activity both for the study population as a whole and comparatively between marker-positive and marker-negative subjects. If the activity in marker-positive subjects is better than in marker-negative subjects in the first stage, the study in the second stage will evaluate marker-positive subjects alone. Otherwise the second-stage study will be an all-comers trial. If this second-stage all-comers trial is not positive and if the activity is much better in marker-positive subjects, then a third-stage trial will be undertaken in marker-positive subjects. Otherwise there will be no further trial.

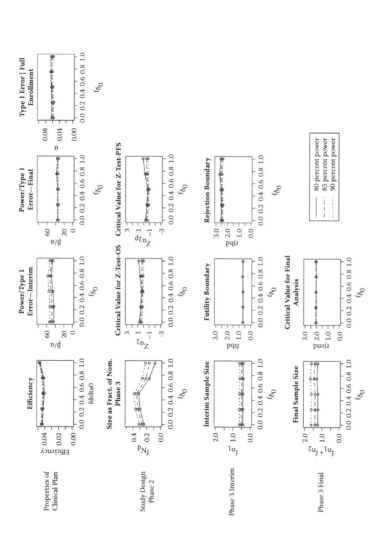

FIGURE 17.5
Properties of dose finding clinical plan, pre-Phase 2 development costs equal zero, probability of no effect on PFS under null equals 0.50.

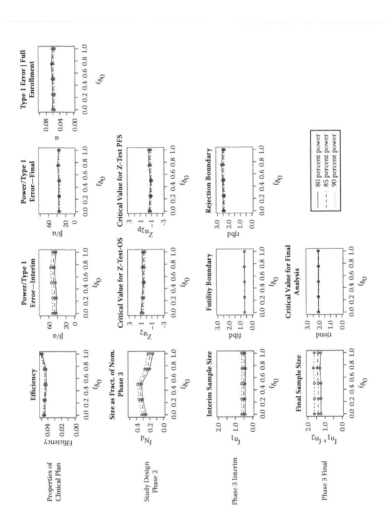

FIGURE 17.6
Properties of dose finding clinical plan, pre-Phase 2 development costs equal zero, probability of no effect on PFS under null equals 0.75.

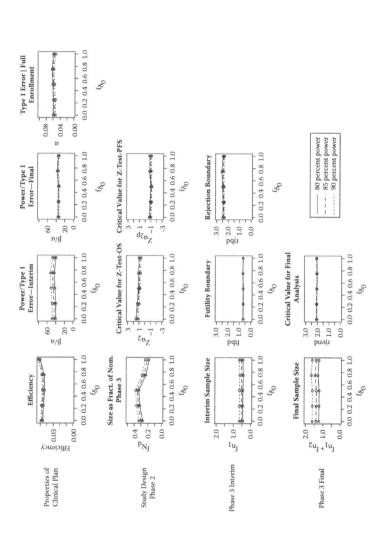

FIGURE 17.7
Properties of dose finding clinical plan, pre-Phase 2 development costs equal zero, probability of no effect on PFS under null equals 0.90.

We can express the efficiency for this three-stage design as follows. Let

$$A = \Phi\left(z_{\alpha_2} - (z_{\alpha_3} - z_\beta) \cdot \left[(f_{\delta^+} - f_{\delta^-}) \cdot \sqrt{\frac{f_{N^+} \cdot f_{N^-}}{f_{N^+} + f_{N^-}}} \right] \cdot \sqrt{f_{N_2}} \right) \qquad (17.25)$$

$$B = \Phi\left(z_{\alpha_3} - (z_{\alpha_3} - z_\beta) \cdot f_{\delta^+} \right) \qquad (17.26)$$

$$C = \Phi\left(z_{\alpha_3} - (z_{\alpha_3} - z_\beta) \cdot f_{pool} \right) \qquad (17.27)$$

$$D = \Phi\left(z_{\alpha_{3b}} - (z_{\alpha_3} - z_\beta) \cdot \left[(f_{\delta^+} - f_{\delta^-}) \cdot \sqrt{\frac{f_{N^+} \cdot f_{N^-}}{f_{N^+} + f_{N^-}}} \right] \right) \qquad (17.28)$$

$$E = \Phi\left(z_{\alpha_3} - (z_{\alpha_3} - z_\beta) \cdot f_{\delta^+} \cdot \sqrt{f_{N_4}} \right) \qquad (17.29)$$

Here

f_{δ^+} = magnitude of the treatment effect in the marker-positive subjects

f_{δ^-} = magnitude of the treatment effect in the marker-negative subjects

f_{N^+} = proportion of subjects enrolled who are marker positive

f_{N^-} = proportion of subjects enrolled who are marker negative

The quantity A represents the probability that the observed treatment effect in the marker-positive subjects is statistically greater than the observed treatment effect in the marker-negative subjects at the α_2 level of significance in Phase 2. B is the probability that a Phase 3 trial in marker-positive subjects is positive. C represents the probability that an all-comers Phase 3 trial is positive. And finally, D represents the probability that a Phase 3 trial detects a statistically significant difference in the treatment effect between marker-positive and marker-negative subjects at the α_{3b} level of significance and E represents the probability that the third-stage trial of marker-positive subjects is positive.

Using this notation, we can write the efficiency of this clinical development plan as

$$\text{Efficiency} = \frac{p \cdot (A \cdot B + (1-A) \cdot [C + (1-C) \cdot D \cdot E])}{N \cdot \{1 + f_{N_2} + 1 + p \cdot (1-A) \cdot (1-C) \cdot D \cdot f_{N_4} + (1-p) \cdot (1-\alpha_2) \cdot (1-\alpha_3) \cdot \alpha_{3b} \cdot f_{N_4}\}}$$

$$(17.30)$$

Table 17.1 describes how we treat all the parameters involved in this expression for efficiency.

Figures 17.8, 17.9, and 17.10 present the results of maximizing efficiency as a function of the treatment effect in the marker-negative subjects. The strategy that maximizes the minimum efficiency for values of f_{δ^+} equal to 0.75, 1, and 1.33, and values of f_{δ^-} ranging from 0 to 1 is presented as well as the strategy that maximizes efficiency at each specific combination of f_{δ^+} and f_{δ^-}, treatment effects in the marker-positive and marker-negative subjects, respectively. Figure 17.8 displays the results when the treatment effect in marker positive subjects corresponds to $f_{\delta^+} = 0.75$, Figure 17.9 shows the results when the treatment effect is $f_{\delta^+} = 1.0$, and Figure 17.10 shows the results when $f_{\delta^+} = 1.33$.

The optimization of the three-stage clinical plan at each combination of f_{δ^+} and f_{δ^-} described here results in parameter values for α_2 close to 1 and for f_{N_2} close to the lower limit 0.10. These solutions can be interepreted as suggesting that the way to optimize efficiency in most circumstances is to not do the Phase 2 screening trial and proceed directly to a Phase 3 type trial in marker-positive subjects. The case where this is not true is an important case, namely, when there is activity in marker-negative subjects greater than but comparable to the activity in marker positive subjects. Since we may want a clinical strategy that performs well in either of these circumstances, we identified values for the parameters that maximize the minimum efficiency over both of these scenarios. The strategy identified that maximizes the minimum efficiency over these possible circumstances indicates that the Phase 2 trial should enroll subjects corresponding to $f_{N_2} = 0.1$ and test at $\alpha_2 = 0.50$. If this test in Phase 2 comparing the treatment effect in marker-positive subjects with marker-negative subjects rejects the null that there is not a difference in the treatment effects, then

TABLE 17.1

Summary of Model Parameters

z_{α_2}	Model fit over range 0.1 to 0.99
z_{α_3}	0.025
$z_{\alpha_{3b}}$	Model fit over range 0.025 to 0.9
z_β	0.80
f_{δ^+}	Set 0.75, 1.00, 1.33
f_{δ^-}	Set range from 0.1 to 1
f_{N^+}	Set at 0.5
f_{N^-}	Set at 0.5
f_{N_2}	Model fit > 0.1
f_{N_4}	Model fit > 1.0

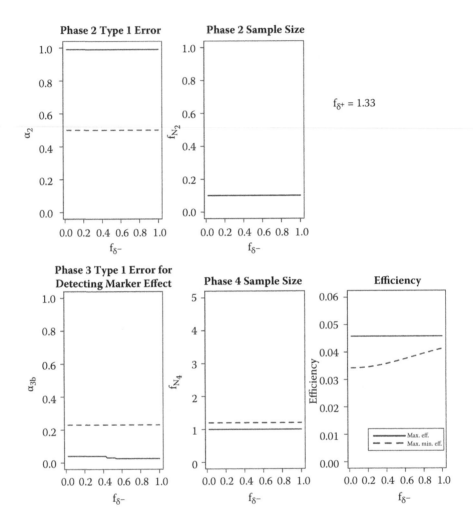

FIGURE 17.8
Three-stage clinical plan to assess the treatment effect in all subjects and marker positive subjects, $f_{\delta^+} = 1.00$.

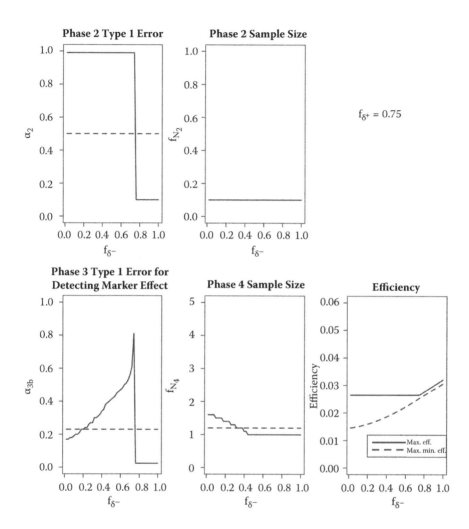

FIGURE 17.9
Three-stage clinical plan to assess the treatment effect in all subjects and marker positive subjects, $f_{\delta^+} = 0.75$.

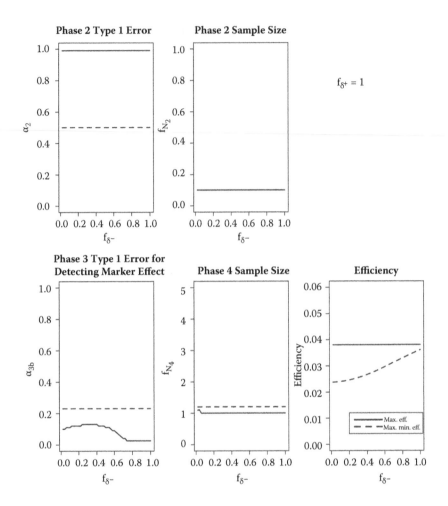

FIGURE 17.10
Three-stage clinical plan to assess the treatment effect in all subjects and marker positive subjects, $f_{\delta^+} = 1.33$.

we proceed to do a Phase 3 trial in marker-positive subjects. If the Phase 2 test fails to reject, then we proceed to do a Phase 3 trial in all subjects. This Phase 3 trial tests to see if there is a treatment effect in all subjects. If there is not a treatment effect in all subjects, then a test is undertaken at $\alpha_{3b} = 0.22$ to see if the treatment effect is greater in marker-positive than in marker-negative subjects. If so, then a second Phase 3 trial in marker positive subjects alone is undertaken with a sample size 1.2 times the Phase 3 sample size.

Appendix A: Maximize Relative Efficiency

In this appendix, we show that maximizing relative efficiency is necessary for maximizing the number of successful Phase 3 studies subject to a constraint on the number of subjects enrolled.

Let k denote the number of studies being evaluated, B denote the budget constraint, and C the cost of a Phase 3 program. Then the solution to maximizing the number of positive Phase 3 trials from an active drug subject to a budget constraint can be obtained with Lagrange multipliers as follows:

$$l = k \cdot p \cdot \Phi\left(z_{\alpha_2} - \left[z_{\alpha_3} - z_\beta\right] \cdot f_\delta \cdot \sqrt{f_N}\right) \cdot \Phi\left(z_{\alpha_3} - \left[z_{\alpha_3} - z_\beta\right] \cdot f_\delta\right)$$
$$+ \lambda \cdot \left[k \cdot f_{N.} \cdot C + k \cdot \left\{p \cdot \Phi\left(z_{\alpha_2} - \left[z_{\alpha_3} - z_\beta\right] \cdot f_\delta \cdot \sqrt{f_N}\right) + (1-p) \cdot \alpha_2\right\} \cdot C - B\right]$$

(A.1)

Taking partials with respect to k, α_2, and f_N, and setting them equal to zero yields the following three equations:

$$\lambda = \frac{p \cdot \Phi\left(z_{\alpha_2} - \left[z_{\alpha_3} - z_\beta\right] \cdot f_\delta \cdot \sqrt{f_N}\right) \cdot \Phi\left(z_{\alpha_3} - \left[z_{\alpha_3} - z_\beta\right] \cdot f_\delta\right)}{C \cdot \left[f_N + p \cdot \Phi\left(z_{\alpha_2} - \left[z_{\alpha_3} - z_\beta\right] \cdot f_\delta \cdot \sqrt{f_N}\right) + (1-p) \cdot \alpha_2\right]}$$

(A.2)

$$\lambda = \frac{p \cdot \phi\left(z_{\alpha_2} - \left[z_{\alpha_3} - z_\beta\right] \cdot f_\delta \cdot \sqrt{f_N}\right) \cdot z'_{\alpha_2} \cdot \Phi\left(z_{\alpha_3} - \left[z_{\alpha_3} - z_\beta\right] \cdot f_\delta\right)}{C \cdot \left[p \cdot \phi\left(z_{\alpha_2} - \left[z_{\alpha_3} - z_\beta\right] \cdot f_\delta \cdot \sqrt{f_N}\right) \cdot z'_{\alpha_2} + (1-p)\right]}$$

(A.3)

$$\lambda = \frac{p \cdot \phi\left(z_{\alpha_2} - \left[z_{\alpha_3} - z_\beta\right] \cdot f_\delta \cdot \sqrt{f_N}\right) \cdot (-1) \cdot \left[z_{\alpha_3} - z_\beta\right] \cdot 1/2 \cdot f_N^{-1/2} \cdot \Phi\left(z_{\alpha_3} - \left[z_{\alpha_3} - z_\beta\right] \cdot f_\delta\right)}{C \cdot \left[1 + p \cdot \phi\left(z_{\alpha_2} - \left[z_{\alpha_3} - z_\beta\right] \cdot f_\delta \cdot \sqrt{f_N}\right) \cdot (-1) \cdot \left[z_{\alpha_3} - z_\beta\right] \cdot 1/2 \cdot f_N^{-1/2}\right]}$$

(A.4)

The efficiency of a Phase 2/3 program is the ratio of the probability of a successful Phase 3 trial to the expected number of subjects enrolled. This can be factored into the efficiency of a Phase 3 trial alone times the relative efficiency:

$$\frac{p \cdot \Phi\left(z_{\alpha_3} - \left[z_{\alpha_3} - z_\beta\right] \cdot f_\delta\right)}{N} \cdot \frac{\Phi\left(z_{\alpha_2} - \left[z_{\alpha_3} - z_\beta\right] \cdot f_\delta \cdot \sqrt{f_N}\right)}{p \cdot \Phi\left(z_{\alpha_2} - \left[z_{\alpha_3} - z_\beta\right] \cdot f_\delta \cdot \sqrt{f_N}\right) + (1-p) \cdot \alpha_2 + f_N}$$

(A.5)

Taking the derivative of the relative efficiency with respect to α_2 leads to

$$\left[p \cdot \Phi\left(z_{\alpha_2}+..\right)+(1-p)\cdot \alpha_2 + f_N\right]\cdot \phi\left(z_{\alpha_2}+..\right)\cdot z'_{\alpha_2}$$
$$-\Phi\left(z_{\alpha_2}+..\right)\cdot\left[p \cdot \phi\left(z_{\alpha_2}+...\right)\cdot z'_{\alpha_2}+(1-p)\right]=0$$

(A.6)

or

$$\left[(1-p)\cdot \alpha_2 + f_N\right]\cdot \phi\left(z_{\alpha_2}+..\right)\cdot z'_{\alpha_2} - \Phi\left(z_{\alpha_2}+..\right)\cdot(1-p)=0 \qquad (A.7)$$

Now from Equations (A.1) and (A.2) we have

$$\frac{p \cdot \Phi\left(z_{\alpha_2}-\left[z_{\alpha_3}-z_\beta\right]\cdot f_\delta \cdot \sqrt{f_N}\right)\cdot \Phi\left(z_{\alpha_3}-\left[z_{\alpha_3}-z_\beta\right]\cdot f_\delta\right)}{C\cdot\left[f_N + p \cdot \Phi\left(z_{\alpha_2}-\left[z_{\alpha_3}-z_\beta\right]\cdot f_\delta \cdot \sqrt{f_N}\right)+(1-p)\cdot \alpha_2\right]}$$
$$=\frac{p \cdot \phi\left(z_{\alpha_2}-\left[z_{\alpha_3}-z_\beta\right]\cdot f_\delta \cdot \sqrt{f_N}\right)\cdot z'_{\alpha_2}\cdot \Phi\left(z_{\alpha_3}-\left[z_{\alpha_3}-z_\beta\right]\cdot f_\delta\right)}{C\cdot\left[p \cdot \phi\left(z_{\alpha_2}-\left[z_{\alpha_3}-z_\beta\right]\cdot f_\delta \cdot \sqrt{f_N}\right)\cdot z'_{\alpha_2}+(1-p)\right]}$$

(A.8)

$$\frac{\Phi\left(z_{\alpha_2}-\left[z_{\alpha_3}-z_\beta\right]\cdot f_\delta \cdot \sqrt{f_N}\right)}{\left[f_N + p \cdot \Phi\left(z_{\alpha_2}-\left[z_{\alpha_3}-z_\beta\right]\cdot f_\delta \cdot \sqrt{f_N}\right)+(1-p)\cdot \alpha_2\right]}$$
$$=\frac{\phi\left(z_{\alpha_2}-\left[z_{\alpha_3}-z_\beta\right]\cdot f_\delta \cdot \sqrt{f_N}\right)\cdot z'_{\alpha_2}}{\left[p \cdot \phi\left(z_{\alpha_2}-\left[z_{\alpha_3}-z_\beta\right]\cdot f_\delta \cdot \sqrt{f_N}\right)\cdot z'_{\alpha_2}+(1-p)\right]}$$

(A.9)

$$\Phi\left(z_{\alpha_2}+..\right)\cdot\left[p \cdot \phi\left(z_{\alpha_2}+..\right)\cdot z'_{\alpha_2}+(1-p)\right]$$
$$=\left[f_N + p \cdot \Phi\left(z_{\alpha_2}+..\right)+(1-p)\cdot \alpha_2\right]\cdot \phi\left(z_{\alpha_2}+..\right)\cdot z'_{\alpha_2}$$

(A.10)

and finally

$$\Phi\left(z_{\alpha_2}+..\right)\cdot(1-p)=\left[(1-p)\cdot \alpha_2 + f_N\right]\cdot \phi\left(z_{\alpha_2}+..\right)\cdot z'_{\alpha_2} \qquad (A.11)$$

Thus, maximizing the number of positive Phase 3 trials from an active drug with respect to α_2 subject to a budget constraint implies that the relative efficiency with respect to α_2 is maximized. Similarly, taking the derivative of the relative efficiency with respect to f_N results in an equation that Equations (A.1) and (A.3) imply must be true. Thus, maximizing the number of successful Phase 3 trials with respect to f_N subject to a budget constraint implies that the relative efficiency is maximized with respect to f_N as well.

Appendix B: An Essentially Complete Class of Phase 2 Screening Trials

Here, we develop an algorithm for calculating the essentially complete class of Phase 2 screening trials. Recall that the relative efficiency is defined as

$RE(\alpha_2, f_N, f_\delta)$

$$= \frac{\Phi\left(z_{\alpha_2} - \left[z_{\alpha_3} - z_\beta\right] \cdot f_\delta \cdot \sqrt{f_N}\right)}{\left[p \cdot \Phi\left(z_{\alpha_2} - \left[z_{\alpha_3} - z_\beta\right] \cdot f_\delta \cdot \sqrt{f_N}\right) + (1-p) \cdot \alpha_2 + f_N + C/N\right] \cdot N/(C+N}$$

(B.1)

By Wald's (1947) theorem, an essentially complete class of Phase 2 screening trials is comprised of all Phase 2 screening trials (α_2, f_N), which maximize

$$\int RE(\alpha_2, f_N, f_\delta) \cdot g(f_\delta) \cdot df_\delta$$

(B.2)

for some prior $g(f_\delta)$. So the following two equations must be satisfied for some $g(f_\delta)$ if (α_2, f_N) is in the essentially complete class

$$\frac{\partial}{\partial \alpha_2} \int RE(\alpha_2, f_N, f_\delta) \cdot g(f_\delta) \cdot df_\delta = 0$$

(B.3)

$$\frac{\partial}{\partial f_N} \int RE(\alpha_2, f_N, f_\delta) \cdot g(f_\delta) \cdot df_\delta = 0$$

(B.4)

Equation (B.3) implies

$$\int \frac{\left[(1-p) \cdot \alpha_2 + f_N + C/N\right] \cdot \phi(a) \cdot \dfrac{\partial z_{\alpha_2}}{\partial \alpha_2} - \Phi(a) \cdot (1-p)}{\left[p \cdot \Phi(a) + (1-p) \cdot \alpha_2 + f_N + C/N\right]^2} \cdot g(f_\delta) \cdot df_\delta = 0 \quad (B.5)$$

where $a = z_{\alpha_2} - \left[z_{\alpha_3} - z_\beta\right] \cdot f_\delta \cdot \sqrt{f_N}$. Further, we can rewrite Equation (B.5) as

$$\left[(1-p) \cdot \alpha_2 + f_N + C/N\right] \cdot \frac{1}{\phi(z_{\alpha_2})} \cdot x_1 - (1-p) = 0$$

(B.6)

where

$$x_1 = \frac{\displaystyle\int \frac{\phi(a) \cdot g(f_\delta) \cdot df_\delta}{\left[p \cdot \Phi(a) + (1-p)\alpha_2 + f_N + C/N\right]^2}}{\displaystyle\int \frac{\Phi(a) \cdot g(f_\delta) \cdot df_\delta}{\left[p \cdot \Phi(a) + (1-p)\alpha_2 + f_N + C/N\right]^2}} \tag{B.7}$$

If we take x_1 as fixed in this equation with

$$x_1 < \frac{\phi(z_{\alpha_2})}{\dfrac{C/N}{1-p} + \alpha_2} \tag{B.8}$$

we can solve for f_N as

$$f_N = (1-p)\left[\frac{\phi(z_{\alpha_2})}{x_1} - \alpha_2\right] - C/N \tag{B.9}$$

Similarly, using Equation (B.4) leads to

$$\left[(1-p)\cdot\alpha_2 + f_N + C/N\right]\cdot(-1)\cdot\left[z_{\alpha_3} - z_\beta\right]\cdot(1/2)\cdot f_N^{-1/2}\cdot x_2 - 1 = 0 \tag{B.10}$$

where

$$x_2 = \frac{\displaystyle\int \frac{\phi(a) \cdot f_\delta \cdot g(f_\delta) \cdot df_\delta}{\left[p \cdot \Phi(a) + (1-p)\alpha_2 + f_N + C/N\right]^2}}{\displaystyle\int \frac{\Phi(a) \cdot g(f_\delta) \cdot df_\delta}{\left[p \cdot \Phi(a) + (1-p)\alpha_2 + f_N + C/N\right]^2}} \tag{B.11}$$

Solving for x_2 produces

$$x_2 = \frac{(-2)\cdot f_N^{1/2}}{\left[\alpha_2\cdot(1-p) + f_N + C/N\right]\cdot\left(z_{\alpha_3} - z_\beta\right)} \tag{B.12}$$

If x_2 as solved for above lies between

$$\min_{g(f_\delta)} \frac{\displaystyle\int \frac{\phi(a) \cdot f_\delta \cdot g(f_\delta) \cdot df_\delta}{\left[p \cdot \Phi(a) + (1-p)\alpha_2 + f_N + C/N\right]^2}}{\displaystyle\int \frac{\Phi(a) \cdot g(f_\delta) \cdot df_\delta}{\left[p \cdot \Phi(a) + (1-p)\alpha_2 + f_N + C/N\right]^2}} \tag{B.13}$$

and

$$\max_{g(f_\delta)} \frac{\displaystyle\int \frac{\phi(a) \cdot f_\delta \cdot g(f_\delta) \cdot df_\delta}{\left[p \cdot \Phi(a) + (1-p)\alpha_2 + f_N + C/N\right]^2}}{\displaystyle\int \frac{\Phi(a) \cdot g(f_\delta) \cdot df_\delta}{\left[p \cdot \Phi(a) + (1-p)\alpha_2 + f_N + C/N\right]^2}} \tag{B.14}$$

where $g(f_\delta)$ satisfies

$$\frac{\displaystyle\int \frac{\phi(a)\cdot g(f_\delta)\cdot df_\delta}{\left[p\cdot\Phi(a)+(1-p)\alpha_2+f_N+C/N\right]^2}}{\displaystyle\int \frac{\Phi(a)\cdot g(f_\delta)\cdot df_\delta}{\left[p\cdot\Phi(a)+(1-p)\alpha_2+f_N+C/N\right]^2}} = x_1 \tag{B.15}$$

then α_2, f_N is a member of an essentially complete class of Phase 2 screening trials.

Now let x_1 be fixed. We claim that the minimum and maximum in Equation (B.13) and Equation (B.14) over all $g(f_\delta)$ can be determined from the minimum and maximum over all two point priors. To see this, suppose that there is a continuous prior $g(f_\delta)$ that maximizes x_2 subject to the constraint $x_1 = D$. Let h represent a two point prior with support on δ_1 and δ_2 that maximizes x_2 subject to the constraint $x_1 = D$ among all two point priors. Create a new prior $w(f_\delta)$ as follows.

Let f_{δ_0} be such that

$$\phi(a(f_{\delta_0}))/\Phi(a(f_{\delta_0})) = x_1 \tag{B.16}$$

Let f_{δ_A} be fixed with $f_{\delta_A} < f_{\delta_0}$ and let f_{δ_B} be such that $f_{\delta_0} < f_{\delta_B}$ and

$$\frac{\displaystyle\frac{\phi(f_{\delta_A})\cdot h(f_{\delta_1})}{\left[p\cdot\Phi(a[f_{\delta_A}])+(1-p)\alpha_2+f_N+C/N\right]^2}+\frac{\phi(f_{\delta_B})\cdot h(f_{\delta_2})}{\left[p\cdot\Phi(a[f_{\delta_B}])+(1-p)\alpha_2+f_N+C/N\right]^2}}{\displaystyle\frac{\Phi(f_{\delta_A})\cdot h(f_{\delta_1})}{\left[p\cdot\Phi(a[f_{\delta_A}])+(1-p)\alpha_2+f_N+C/N\right]^2}+\frac{\Phi(f_{\delta_B})\cdot h(f_{\delta_2})}{\left[p\cdot\Phi(a[f_{\delta_B}])+(1-p)\alpha_2+f_N+C/N\right]^2}} = x_1 \tag{B.17}$$

Equation (B.17) defines a relationship between f_{δ_A} and f_{δ_B}, namely, $f_{\delta_B} = u(f_{\delta_A})$. u is continuous and monotone decreasing since $\varphi(x)/\Phi(x)$ is continuous and monotone decreasing.

Define $w(f_\delta)$ as

$$w(f_\delta) = g(f_\delta) - r\cdot\left\{h(f_{\delta_1})\cdot I_{S_-}(f_\delta)+\frac{h(f_{\delta_2})}{|df_{\delta_B}/df_{\delta_A}|}\cdot I_{S_+}(f_\delta)\right\}$$
$$+ h(f_{\delta_1})\cdot I_{f_{\delta_1}}(f_\delta)+h(f_{\delta_2})\cdot I_{f_{\delta_2}}(f_\delta) \tag{B.18}$$

where $S_- = \{f_\delta : \gamma_1 < f_\delta < \gamma_2 \quad \text{where } \gamma_1 < \gamma_2 < f_{\delta_0}\}$ and $S_+ = u(S_-)$. The second term in the definition of $w(f_\delta)$ represents a continuous decrement from $g(f_\delta)$, and the third term represents a discrete increment. The constants γ_1 and γ_2 are chosen so that

$$\frac{\displaystyle\int_{S_- \cup S_+} \frac{\phi(a) \cdot f_\delta \cdot g(f_\delta) \cdot df_\delta}{\left[p \cdot \Phi(a) + (1-p)\alpha_2 + f_N + C/N \right]^2}}{\displaystyle\int_{S_- \cup S_+} \frac{\Phi(a) \cdot g(f_\delta) \cdot df_\delta}{\left[p \cdot \Phi(a) + (1-p)\alpha_2 + f_N + C/N \right]^2}} \le x_2 \tag{B.19}$$

If no such γ_1 and γ_2 exist, then

$$\frac{\displaystyle\int_R \frac{\phi(a) \cdot f_\delta \cdot g(f_\delta) \cdot df_\delta}{\left[p \cdot \Phi(a) + (1-p)\alpha_2 + f_N + C/N \right]^2}}{\displaystyle\int_R \frac{\Phi(a) \cdot g(f_\delta) \cdot df_\delta}{\left[p \cdot \Phi(a) + (1-p)\alpha_2 + f_N + C/N \right]^2}} > x_2 \tag{B.20}$$

which contradicts our assumption about g in Equation (B.11). r is chosen so that

$$r \cdot \int_0^\infty \left[h(f_{\delta_1}) \cdot I_{S_-}\left(f_\delta\right) + \frac{h(f_{\delta_2})}{df_{\delta_B}/df_{\delta_A}} \cdot I_{S_+}\left(f_\delta\right) \right] \cdot df_\delta = h(f_{\delta_1}) + h(f_{\delta_2}) \tag{B.21}$$

and

$$g(f_\delta) - r \cdot \left\{ h(f_{\delta_1}) \cdot I_{S_-}\left(f_\delta\right) + \frac{h(f_{\delta_2})}{df_{\delta_B}/df_{\delta_A}} \cdot I_{S_+}\left(f_\delta\right) \right\} > 0 \tag{B.22}$$

Now by assumption we have that

$$\frac{\displaystyle\int \frac{\phi(a[f_\delta]) \cdot g(f_\delta)}{\left\{ p \cdot \Phi(a[f_\delta]) + (1-p)\alpha_2 + f_N + C/N \right\}^2} \cdot df_\delta}{\displaystyle\int \frac{\Phi(a[f_\delta]) \cdot g(f_\delta)}{\left\{ p \cdot \Phi(a[f_\delta]) + (1-p)\alpha_2 + f_N + C/N \right\}^2} \cdot df_\delta} = x_1 \tag{B.23}$$

and

$$\frac{\displaystyle\int \frac{\phi(a[f_\delta]) \cdot d\left(h(f_{\delta_1}) \cdot I_{\{f_{\delta_1}\}}(f_\delta) + h(f_{\delta_2}) \cdot I_{\{f_{\delta_2}\}}(f_\delta) \right)}{\left\{ p \cdot \Phi(a[f_\delta]) + (1-p)\alpha_2 + f_N + C/N \right\}^2} \cdot df_\delta}{\displaystyle\int \frac{\Phi(a[f_\delta]) \cdot d\left(h(f_{\delta_1}) \cdot I_{\{f_{\delta_1}\}}(f_\delta) + h(f_{\delta_2}) \cdot I_{\{f_{\delta_2}\}}(f_\delta) \right)}{\left\{ p \cdot \Phi(a[f_\delta]) + (1-p)\alpha_2 + f_N + C/N \right\}^2} \cdot df_\delta} = x_1 \tag{B.24}$$

Further, by the way f_{δ_B} is implicitly defined in Equation (B.17)

$$\frac{\int \frac{\phi(a[f_\delta]) \cdot \left(h(f_{\delta_1}) \cdot I_{\{S_-\}}(f_\delta) + \frac{h(f_{\delta_2})}{df_{\delta_B} / df_{\delta_A}} \cdot I_{\{S_+\}}(f_\delta) \right) \cdot df_\delta}{\left\{ p \cdot \Phi(a[f_\delta]) + (1-p)\alpha_2 + f_N + C/N \right\}^2}}{\int \frac{\Phi(a[f_\delta]) \cdot \left(h(f_{\delta_1}) \cdot I_{\{S_-\}}(f_\delta) + \frac{h(f_{\delta_2})}{df_{\delta_B} / df_{\delta_A}} \cdot I_{\{S_+\}}(f_\delta) \right) \cdot df_\delta}{\left\{ p \cdot \Phi(a[f_\delta]) + (1-p)\alpha_2 + f_N + C/N \right\}^2}} = x_1 \qquad \text{(B.25)}$$

To see this let $\{s_1, s_2, \ldots s_k\}$ be a partition of S_-. Then by the monotonicity of $u()$, $\{u(s_1), u(s_2), \ldots u(s_k)\}$ is also a partition of S_+ and by the continuity of $u()$, $u(s_j) - u(s_{j-1}) \to 0$ as $s_j - s_{j-1} \to 0$. Further

$$\frac{h(f_{\delta_1}) \cdot (s_j - s_{j-1})}{\frac{h(f_{\delta_2})}{df_{\delta_B} / df_{\delta_A}} \cdot \left[u(s_j) - u(s_{j-1}) \right]} = \frac{h(f_{\delta_1}) \cdot (s_j - s_{j-1}) \cdot \frac{du(s)}{ds}}{h(f_{\delta_2}) \cdot \left[u(s_j) - u(s_{j-1}) \right]} \approx \frac{h(f_{\delta_1})}{h(f_{\delta_2})} \qquad \text{(B.26)}$$

So, for each term in the Riemann sum for the integrals in Equation (B.25), there exists a real k such that

$$h(f_{\delta_1}) \cdot (s_j - s_{j-1}) \approx h(f_{\delta_1}) \cdot k_j \qquad \text{(B.27)}$$

and

$$\frac{h(f_{\delta_2})}{df_{\delta_B} / df_{\delta_A}} \cdot \left[u(s_j) - u(s_{j-1}) \right] \approx h(f_{\delta_2}) \cdot k_j \qquad \text{(B.28)}$$

So

$$\frac{\int \phi(a[f_\delta]) \cdot \frac{\left(h(f_{\delta_1}) \cdot I_{\{S_-\}}(f_\delta) + \frac{h(f_{\delta_2})}{df_{\delta_B} / df_{\delta_A}} \cdot I_{\{S_+\}}(f_\delta) \right)}{\left\{ p \cdot \Phi(a[f_\delta]) + (1-p)\alpha_2 + f_N + C/N \right\}^2} \cdot df_\delta}{\int \Phi(a[f_\delta]) \cdot \frac{\left(h(f_{\delta_1}) \cdot I_{\{S_-\}}(f_\delta) + \frac{h(f_{\delta_2})}{df_{\delta_B} / df_{\delta_A}} \cdot I_{\{S_+\}}(f_\delta) \right)}{\left\{ p \cdot \Phi(a[f_\delta]) + (1-p)\alpha_2 + f_N + C/N \right\}^2} \cdot df_\delta} = \qquad \text{(B.29)}$$

$$\frac{\displaystyle\sum_j \left(\frac{\phi(a[s_j]) \cdot h(f_{\delta_1}) \cdot (s_j - s_{j-1})}{\left\{ p \cdot \Phi(a[s_j]) + (1-p)\alpha_2 + \ldots \right\}^2} + \frac{\phi(a[u(s_j)]) \cdot \frac{h(f_{\delta_2})}{df_{\delta_B} / df_{\delta_A}} \cdot \left[u(s_j) - u(s_{j-1}) \right]}{\left\{ p \cdot \Phi(a[u(s_j)]) + (1-p)\alpha_2 + \ldots \right\}^2} \right)}{\displaystyle\sum_j \left(\frac{\Phi(a[s_j]) \cdot h(f_{\delta_1}) \cdot (s_j - s_{j-1})}{\left\{ p \cdot \Phi(a[s_j]) + (1-p)\alpha_2 + \ldots \right\}^2} + \frac{\Phi(a[u(s_j)]) \cdot \frac{h(f_{\delta_2})}{df_{\delta_B} / df_{\delta_A}} \cdot \left[u(s_j) - u(s_{j-1}) \right]}{\left\{ p \cdot \Phi(a[u(s_j)]) + (1-p)\alpha_2 + \ldots \right\}^2} \right)} =$$

$$\text{(B.30)}$$

$$\frac{\displaystyle\sum_{j}\left(\frac{\phi(a[s_j])\cdot h(f_{\delta_1})\cdot k_j}{\left\{p\cdot\Phi(a[s_j])+(1-p)\alpha_2+\ldots\right\}^2}+\frac{\phi(a[u(s_j)])\cdot h(f_{\delta_2})\cdot k_j}{\left\{p\cdot\Phi(a[u(s_j)])+(1-p)\alpha_2+\ldots\right\}^2}\right)}{\displaystyle\sum_{j}\left(\frac{\Phi(a[s_j])\cdot h(f_{\delta_1})\cdot k_j}{\left\{p\cdot\Phi(a[s_j])+(1-p)\alpha_2+\ldots\right\}^2}+\frac{\Phi(a[u(s_j)])\cdot h(f_{\delta_2})\cdot k_j}{\left\{p\cdot\Phi(a[u(s_j)])+(1-p)\alpha_2+\ldots\right\}^2}\right)}=\quad\text{(B.31)}$$

$$\frac{\displaystyle\sum_{j}\left(\frac{\phi(a[s_j])\cdot h(f_{\delta_1})}{\left\{p\cdot\Phi(a[s_j])+(1-p)\alpha_2+\ldots\right\}^2}+\frac{\phi(a[u(s_j)])\cdot h(f_{\delta_2})}{\left\{p\cdot\Phi(a[u(s_j)])+(1-p)\alpha_2+\ldots\right\}^2}\right)}{\displaystyle\sum_{j}\left(\frac{\Phi(a[s_j])\cdot h(f_{\delta_1})}{\left\{p\cdot\Phi(a[s_j])+(1-p)\alpha_2+\ldots\right\}^2}+\frac{\Phi(a[u(s_j)])\cdot h(f_{\delta_2})}{\left\{p\cdot\Phi(a[u(s_j)])+(1-p)\alpha_2+\ldots\right\}^2}\right)}=x_1$$

$$\text{(B.32)}$$

The last expression equals x_1 since the ratio of the two summands is x_1 for each j by Equation (B.17).

Thus, we have that

$$\frac{\displaystyle\int\frac{\phi(a)\cdot dw(f_\delta)}{\left\{p\cdot\Phi(a[f_\delta])+(1-p)\alpha_2+f_N+C/N\right\}^2}}{\displaystyle\int\frac{\Phi(a)\cdot dw(f_\delta)}{\left\{p\cdot\Phi(a[f_\delta])+(1-p)\alpha_2+f_N+C/N\right\}^2}}=x_1 \qquad\text{(B.33)}$$

since

$$\frac{a}{b}=\frac{c}{d}=\frac{e}{f}=x\Rightarrow\frac{a+c+e}{b+d+f}=x \qquad\text{(B.34)}$$

Further

$$\frac{\displaystyle\int\frac{\phi(a[f_\delta])\cdot f_\delta\cdot g(f_\delta)\cdot df_\delta}{\left\{p\cdot\Phi(a[f_\delta])+(1-p)\alpha_2+f_N+C/N\right\}^2}}{\displaystyle\int\frac{\Phi(a[f_\delta])\cdot g(f_\delta)\cdot df_\delta}{\left\{p\cdot\Phi(a[f_\delta])+(1-p)\alpha_2+f_N+C/N\right\}^2}}$$

$$\text{(B.35)}$$

$$<\frac{\displaystyle\int\frac{\phi(a[f_\delta])\cdot f_\delta\cdot w(f_\delta)\cdot df_\delta}{\left\{p\cdot\Phi(a[f_\delta])+(1-p)\alpha_2+f_N+C/N\right\}^2}}{\displaystyle\int\frac{\Phi(a[f_\delta])\cdot w(f_\delta)\cdot df_\delta}{\left\{p\cdot\Phi(a[f_\delta])+(1-p)\alpha_2+f_N+C/N\right\}^2}}$$

since by the definition of h as the two point prior that maximizes the objective function

$$\frac{\int \frac{\phi(a[f_\delta]) \cdot f_\delta \cdot r \cdot \left(h(f_{\delta_1}) \cdot I_{\{S_{\delta_A}\}}(f_\delta) + \frac{h(f_{\delta_2})}{df_{\delta_B} / df_{\delta_A}} \cdot I_{\{S_{\delta_B}\}}(f_\delta) \right) \cdot df_\delta}{\{p \cdot \Phi(a[f_\delta]) + (1-p)\alpha_2 + f_N + C / N\}^2}}{\int \frac{\Phi(a[f_\delta]) \cdot r \cdot \left(h(f_{\delta_1}) \cdot I_{\{S_{\delta_A}\}}(f_\delta) + \frac{h(f_{\delta_2})}{df_{\delta_B} / df_{\delta_A}} \cdot I_{\{S_{\delta_B}\}}(f_\delta) \right) \cdot df_\delta}{\{p \cdot \Phi(a[f_\delta]) + (1-p)\alpha_2 + f_N + C / N\}^2}} = \quad \text{(B.36)}$$

$$\frac{\sum_j \left(\phi(a[s_j]) \cdot s_j \cdot \frac{h(f_{\delta_1})}{\{p \cdot \Phi(a[s_j]+\ldots\}^2} + \phi(a[u(s_j)]) \cdot u(s_j) \cdot \frac{h(f_{\delta_2})}{\{p \cdot \Phi(a[u(s_j)]+\ldots\}^2} \right)}{\sum_j \left(\Phi(a[s_j]) \cdot \frac{h(f_{\delta_1})}{\{p \cdot \Phi(a[s_j]+\ldots\}^2} + \Phi(a[u(s_j)]) \cdot \frac{h(f_{\delta_2})}{\{p \cdot \Phi(a[u(s_j)]+\ldots\}^2} \right)} \leq$$

$$\text{(B.37)}$$

$$\frac{\sum_j \left(\phi(a[f_{\delta_1}]) \cdot f_{\delta_1} \cdot \frac{h(f_{\delta_1})}{\{p \cdot \Phi(a[f_{\delta_1}]+\ldots\}^2} + \phi(a[f_{\delta_2}]) \cdot f_{\delta_2} \cdot \frac{h(f_{\delta_2})}{\{p \cdot \Phi(a[u(f_{\delta_2})]+\ldots\}^2} \right)}{\sum_j \left(\Phi(a[f_{\delta_1}]) \cdot \frac{h(f_{\delta_1})}{\{p \cdot \Phi(a[f_{\delta_1}]+\ldots\}^2} + \Phi(a[f_{\delta_2}]) \cdot \frac{h(f_{\delta_2})}{\{p \cdot \Phi(a[u(f_{\delta_2})]+\ldots\}^2} \right)}$$

$$\text{(B.38)}$$

This last inequality follows since h with support on δ_1 and δ_2 maximizes x_2 subject to the constraint $x_1 = D$ among all two point priors. This inequality implies that

$$\frac{\int \frac{\phi(a) \cdot f_\delta \cdot g(f_\delta) \cdot df_\delta}{\{p \cdot \Phi(a[f_\delta]) + (1-p)\alpha_2 + \ldots\}^2}}{\int \frac{\Phi(a) \cdot g(f_\delta) \cdot df_\delta}{\{p \cdot \Phi(a[f_\delta]) + (1-p)\alpha_2 + \ldots\}^2}} < \frac{\int \frac{\phi(a) \cdot f_\delta \cdot dw(f_\delta)}{\{p \cdot \Phi(a[f_\delta]) + (1-p)\alpha_2 + \ldots\}^2}}{\int \frac{\Phi(a) \cdot dw(f_\delta)}{\{p \cdot \Phi(a[f_\delta]) + (1-p)\alpha_2 + \ldots\}^2}} \quad \text{(B.39)}$$

Therefore, x_2 is not maximized with a continuous prior. Since a similar argument can be applied for any prior that is not a two point prior we conclude that x_2 is maximized with a two point prior.

Figure B.1 shows the Phase 2 trials that comprise an essentially complete class when C/N is 1 and $p = 0.20$. The solid line represents the maximum sample size for a given type 1 error in Phase 2 that yields a Phase 2 screening trial that is not dominated by a Phase 3 trial alone in terms of efficiency. The circles represent Phase 2 screening trials in the essentially complete class.

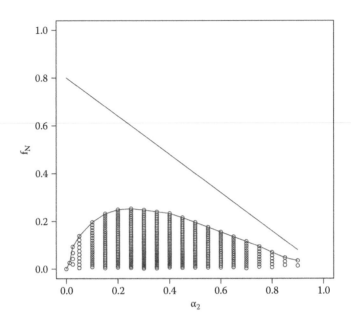

FIGURE B.1
A complete class of Phase 2 designs. $C/N = 1$.

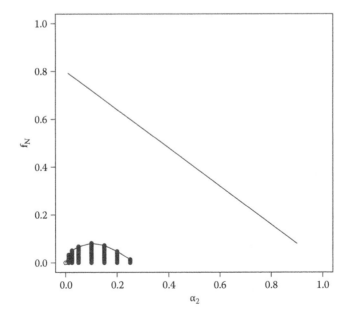

FIGURE B.2
A complete class of Phase 2 designs. $C/N = 0$.

For every Phase 2 screening trial not in this region, there exists a Phase 2 screening trial in the region with relative efficiency at least as great for all values of f_δ. This region immediately yields an upper bound on the sample size of a trial for every level of type 1 error and a range of type 1 errors for every Phase 2 sample size.

Figure B.2 provides the same figure when $C = 0$ and $p = 0.20$. The essentially complete family of Phase 2 designs is smaller (more restricted) in the case where $C/N = 0$. The Phase 2 sample size need be no bigger than 10 percent of the Phase 3 sample size and the one-sided type 1 error should be no bigger than 25 percent.

Reference

Wald, A. 1947. An essentially complete class of admissible decision functions. *Ann Math Stat* 18(4):549–555.

Appendix C: Monotonicity of Power/Type 1 Error

First note that

$$\frac{\beta}{\alpha} = \frac{1 - \Phi\left(z_\alpha - \delta / \sqrt{2 \cdot \sigma^2 / n}\right)}{1 - \Phi(z_\alpha)} \tag{C.1}$$

In terms of the probability of seeing results more extreme than what was observed, X, we have

$$\frac{\beta}{\alpha} = \frac{1 - \Phi\left(X - \delta / \sqrt{2 \cdot \sigma^2 / n}\right)}{1 - \Phi(X)} \tag{C.2}$$

Now

$$\lim_{X \to \infty} \frac{1 - \Phi\left(X - \delta / \sqrt{2 \cdot \sigma^2 / n}\right)}{1 - \Phi(X)} = \lim_{X \to \infty} \frac{\phi\left(X - \delta / \sqrt{2 \cdot \sigma^2 / n}\right)}{\phi(X)} \tag{C.3}$$

$$= \lim_{X \to \infty} \frac{\exp\left[-1/2 \cdot (x - a)^2\right] \cdot (x - a)}{\exp\left[-1/2 \cdot x^2\right] \cdot x} \tag{C.4}$$

$$= \lim_{X \to \infty} \exp\left[xb - 1/2 \cdot a^2\right] \cdot \frac{(x - a)}{x} = \begin{cases} \infty & \text{if } a > 0 \\ 1 & \text{if } a = 0 \\ 0 & \text{if } a < 0 \end{cases} \tag{C.5}$$

So, as X increases the ratio of power to type 1 error increases in the limit to infinity. Further, the ratio is monotonically increasing in X for $\delta > 0$ as shown next.

$$\frac{\partial}{\partial x} \frac{1 - \Phi(x - a)}{1 - \Phi(x)} = \frac{\left\{\frac{1 - \Phi(x - a)}{1 - \Phi(x)} - \frac{\phi(x - a)}{\phi(x)}\right\} \cdot [1 - \Phi(x)] \cdot \phi(x)}{[1 - \Phi(x)]^2} > 0 \tag{C.6}$$

if and only if

$$\frac{1 - \Phi(x - a)}{1 - \Phi(x)} - \frac{\phi(x - a)}{\phi(x)} > 0 \tag{C.7}$$

if and only if

$$\int_x^\infty \frac{\phi(t-a)}{\phi(x-a)} dt > \int_x^\infty \frac{\phi(t)}{\phi(x)} dt \qquad (C.8)$$

If we let

$$f(t, a) = \exp\{-1/2 \cdot [t^2 - 2at + a^2] + 1/2 \cdot [x^2 - 2ax + a^2]\} \qquad (C.9)$$

then,

$$\frac{d}{dt} f(t,a) = -(t-a) \cdot f(t,a) \qquad (C.10)$$

Since $f(x,a) = f(x,0)$ it follows that

$$\left| \frac{d}{dt} f(x,a) \right| < \left| \frac{d}{dt} f(x,0) \right| \qquad (C.11)$$

when $x > a > 0$. Indeed, for any s where $s > a$ and $f(s,a) \le f(s,0)$, we have

$$\left| \frac{d}{dt} f(s,a) \right| < \left| \frac{d}{dt} f(s,0) \right| \qquad (C.12)$$

Thus

$$f(s,a) \ge f(s,0) \quad \text{and} \quad \forall s > a \qquad (C.13)$$

since the derivative is negative and so

$$\int_x^\infty \frac{\phi(t-a)}{\phi(x-a)} dt > \int_x^\infty \frac{\phi(t)}{\phi(x)} dt \qquad (C.14)$$

which implies

$$\frac{\partial}{\partial x} \frac{1-\Phi(x-a)}{1-\Phi(x)} > 0 \qquad (C.15)$$

when $x > a > 0$.

Appendix D: The Log Rank Test Maximizes the Power under Proportional Hazards

In this appendix we review the reasoning that supports the proposition that the log rank test maximizes the power under the assumption of proportional hazards.

Assume that the survival times in the experimental treatment arm, $x_{T,1} \ldots x_{T,n_T}$, and the control arm, $x_{C,1} \ldots x_{C,n_C}$, are exponentially distributed. When there is no censoring the likelihood can be expressed as

$$\lambda_C^{n_C} \exp\left(-\lambda_C \cdot \sum_{i=1}^{n_C} x_{C,i}\right) \cdot \lambda_T^{n_T} \exp\left(-\lambda_T \cdot \sum_{j=1}^{n_T} x_{T,j}\right)$$

$$= \lambda_C^{n_C} \lambda_T^{n_T} \exp\left(-(\lambda_T - \lambda_C) \cdot \sum_{j=1}^{n_T} x_{T,j} - \lambda_C \cdot \left[\sum_{i=1}^{n_C} x_{C,i} + \sum_{j=1}^{n_T} x_{T,j}\right]\right) \quad \text{(D.1)}$$

Note that testing $\lambda_T - \lambda_C = 0$ is the same as testing $\lambda_T / \lambda_C = 1$. Further note that

$\sum_{j=1}^{n_T} x_{T,j} \Big/ \sum_{i=1}^{n_C} x_{C,i}$ is monotonically increasing in $\sum_{j=1}^{n_T} x_{T,j}$ and is independent

of $\sum_{i=1}^{n_C} x_{C,i} + \sum_{j=1}^{n_T} x_{T,j}$ when $\lambda_T / \lambda_C = 1$. Thus the F-test

$$\frac{\sum_{j=1}^{n_T} x_{T,j} / (2 \cdot n_T)}{\sum_{i=1}^{n_C} x_{C,i} / (2 \cdot n_C)} \quad \text{(D.2)}$$

for comparing the hazard ratio of two exponential distributions is the uniformly most powerful unbiased test of $\lambda_T / \lambda_C = 1$ (Lehmann 1959).

If we suppose that there is censoring, then the likelihood can be written as

$$\prod_{i=1}^{n_C}\left\{\left[\lambda_C\exp(-\lambda_C\cdot x_{C,i})\cdot(1-G(x_{C,i}))\right]^{d_{C,i}}\cdot\left[g(y_{C,i})\cdot\exp(-\lambda_{C,i}\cdot y_{C,i})\right]^{1-d_{C,i}}\right\}$$

$$\times\prod_{j=1}^{n_T}\left\{\left[\lambda_T\exp(-\lambda_T\cdot x_{T,j})\cdot(1-G(x_{T,j}))\right]^{d_{T,j}}\cdot\left[g(y_{T,j})\cdot\exp(-\lambda_T\cdot y_{T,j})\right]^{1-d_{T,j}}\right\}$$

$$(D.3)$$

Since terms involving G and g drop out in the likelihood ratio, we can consider the following expression as the likelihood:

$$\exp\left(\begin{array}{l}\left[\log(\lambda_T)-\log(\lambda_C)\right]\cdot\sum_{j=1}^{n_T}d_{T,j}+\log(\lambda_C)\cdot\left[\sum_{i=1}^{n_C}d_{C,i}+\sum_{j=1}^{n_T}d_{T,j}\right]\\[3mm] -\lambda_C\left[\sum_{d_{C_i}=1}x_{C,i}+\sum_{d_{C_i}\neq1}y_{C,i}\right]-\lambda_T\left[\sum_{d_{T_j}=1}x_{T,j}+\sum_{d_{T_j}\neq1}y_{T,j}\right]\end{array}\right)\qquad(D.4)$$

So, the uniformly most powerful test has to be a function of $\sum_{j=1}^{n_T}d_{T,j}$. The statistic

$$\frac{\log\left(\sum_{j=1}^{n_T}d_{T,j}/\left[\sum_{d_{T_j}=1}x_{T,j}+\sum_{d_{T_j}\neq1}y_{T,j}\right]\right)-\log\left(\sum_{i=1}^{n_C}d_{C,i}/\left[\sum_{d_{C_i}=1}x_{C,i}+\sum_{d_{C_i}\neq1}y_{C,i}\right]\right)}{\sqrt{1/\sum_{j=1}^{n_T}d_{T,j}+1/\sum_{i=1}^{n_C}d_{C,i}}}$$

$$(D.5)$$

is a monotone function of $\sum_{j=1}^{n_T}d_{T,j}$ and asymptotically is normally distributed with mean zero and variance one when $\lambda_T/\lambda_C = 1$. Thus for large n this test will be close to a uniformly most powerful unbiased test.

Schoenfeld (1981) derived the asymptotic distribution for the log rank test and determined that the distribution matches the distribution of the F-test when there is no censoring. Further, the asymptotic distribution when there is censoring matches the distribution for the asymptotically most powerful unbiased test identified earlier. The result follows by noting the invariance of the log rank test with respect to monotone transformations of the measurement scale.

References

Lehmann, E.L. 1959. *Testing Statistical Hypotheses*. New York: Wiley.

Schoenfeld, D. 1981. The asymptotic properties of nonparametric tests for comparing survival distributions. *Biometrika* 68(1):316–319.

Appendix E: Approximation of the Log Rank Test

In this appendix we wish to show that $\max_{0<s<T} r(s) = o_p(1)$ for any T with $F_1(T) > 0$ and $F_2(T) > 0$, where from Equations (14.2) through (14.4) (see Chapter 14) we have

$$r(s) = \frac{\bar{Y}_1(s)}{n_1(1-F_1(s))} \cdot \frac{\bar{Y}_2(s)}{n_2(1-F_2(s))} \cdot \frac{n_1(1-F_1(s))+n_2(1-F_2(s))}{\bar{Y}_1(s)+\bar{Y}_2(s)} - 1 \qquad (E.1)$$

First, note that

$$P\left(\sup_{0<s<T} \left| \frac{\bar{Y}_1(s)}{n_1} - [1-F_1(s)] \right| > \varepsilon \right)$$

$$= P\left(\sqrt{n} \sup_{0<s<T} \left| \frac{\bar{Y}_1(s)}{n_1} - [1-F_1(s)] \right| > \sqrt{n}\varepsilon \right) \rightarrow_{n \to \infty} 0 \qquad (E.2)$$

since

$$\sqrt{n} \sup_{0<s<T} \left| \frac{\bar{Y}_1(s)}{n_1} - [1-F_1(s)] \right| \rightarrow_{n \to \infty} \text{Kolmogorov distribution}$$

Further, since

$$\sup_{0<s<T} \left| \frac{\bar{Y}_1(s)}{n_1} - [1-F_1(s)] \right| = \sup_{0<s<T} \left| [1-F_1(s)] \cdot \left(\frac{\bar{Y}_1(s)/n_1}{1-F_1(s)} - 1 \right) \right| \qquad (E.3)$$

$$= \sup_{0<s<T} \left(|1-F_1(s)| \cdot \left| \frac{\bar{Y}_1(s)/n_1}{1-F_1(s)} - 1 \right| \right) \qquad (E.4)$$

$$\geq \left(\min_{0<s<T} |1-F_1(s)| \cdot \sup_{0<s<T} \left| \frac{\bar{Y}_1(s)/n_1}{1-F_1(s)} - 1 \right| \right) \qquad (E.5)$$

$$= \left(k \cdot \sup_{0<s<T} \left| \frac{\bar{Y}_1(s)/n_1}{1-F_1(s)} - 1 \right| \right) \qquad (E.6)$$

we have that

$$P\left(\sup_{0<s<T}\left|\frac{\bar{Y}_1(s)/n_1}{1-F_1(s)}-1\right|>\varepsilon\right)<P\left(\sup_{0<s<T}\left|\frac{\bar{Y}_1(s)}{n_1}-[1-F_1(s)]\right|>k\cdot\varepsilon\right)\to_{n\to\infty}0$$

$$(E.7)$$

Since ε is arbitrary we have that $\dfrac{\bar{Y}_1(s)/n_1}{1-F_1(s)}$ converges to 1 uniformly in

probability over $[0,T]$. Similarly, $\dfrac{\bar{Y}_2(s)}{n_2(1-F_2(s))}$ and $\dfrac{n_1(1-F_1(s))+n_2(1-F_2(s))}{\bar{Y}_1(s)+\bar{Y}_2(s)}$

converge to 1 uniformly in probability over $[0,T]$. Therefore, $r(s)$ converges to 1 uniformly in probability over $[0,T]$.

Under censoring

$$r(s)=\frac{\bar{Y}_1(s)}{n_1(1-F_1(s)\cdot G(s))}\cdot\frac{\bar{Y}_2(s)}{n_2(1-F_2(s)\cdot G(s))}$$

$$\cdot\frac{n_1(1-F_1(s)\cdot G(s))+n_2(1-F_2(s)\cdot G(s))}{\bar{Y}_1(s)+\bar{Y}_2(s)}-1$$

$$(E.8)$$

and a similar argument applies to show that $\max_s r(s) = o_p(1)$.

Index

Printed and bound by CPI Group (UK) Ltd, Croydon, CR0 4YY

21/10/2024

01777109-0002